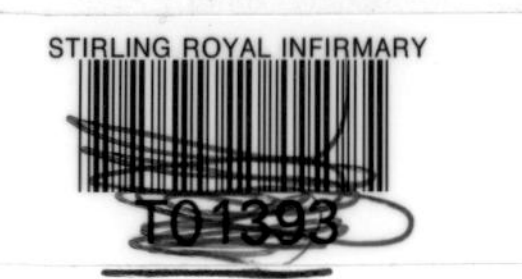
STIRLING ROYAL INFIRMARY
T01393

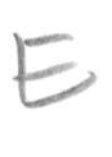

D0335117

# Drugs and Pregnancy

# Drugs and Pregnancy

## HUMAN TERATOGENESIS AND RELATED PROBLEMS

---

Edited by

**D. F. Hawkins**

PhD, DSc, MB, BS(Lond), MD(Mass), FRCOG, FACOG

Professor of Obstetric Therapeutics, Institute of Obstetrics and Gynaecology;
Consultant Obstetrician and Gynaecologist, Hammersmith Hospital, London

CHURCHILL LIVINGSTONE
EDINBURGH LONDON MELBOURNE AND NEW YORK 1983

CHURCHILL LIVINGSTONE
Medical Division of Longman Group Limited

Distributed in the United States of America by
Churchill Livingstone Inc., 1560 Broadway, New York,
N.Y. 10036, and by associated companies, branches
and representatives throughout the world.



First published 1983

ISBN 0 443 02466 9

British Library Catatoguing in Publication Data
Drugs and pregnancy.
1. Fetus, Effects of Drugs on — Congresses
2. Teratogenic agents — Congresses
I. Hawkins, D.F.
618.3′2 RG627

Library of Congress Cataloging in Publication Data
Main entry under title:
Drugs and pregnancy.
Based on papers presented at a meeting held by the Institute of Obstetrics and Gynaecology on 30 May 1980.
Includes bibliographical references and index.
1. Fetus — Effects of drugs on — Congresses.
2. Abnormalities, Human — Etiology — Congresses.
3. Pregnancy, Complications of — Congresses.
I. Hawkins, D. F. (Denis Frank) II. University of London. Institute of Obstetrics and Gynaecology.
[DNLM: 1. Drug therapy — In pregnancy —Congresses.
2. Abnormalities, Drug-Induced — Congresses. QS 679 D794 1980]
RG627.6.D79D795 1983 618.3′2 82-17813

Printed in Great Britain by
Butler & Tanner Ltd, Frome and London

# Preface

Drugs are not a common cause of congenital abnormality, but they are a very important factor, because their ill-effects are potentially preventable by careful therapeutics.

We have been gravely concerned by the plight of the practising clinician with respect to the problem of using drugs in pregnancy. He is assailed on the one hand by the self-protective proclamations of the pharmaceutical houses and the governmental agencies, on the other by the practical needs of his patients for whom he must prescribe treatment. At the same time he is under the threat that one of those very patients, who may have an abnormal baby for a totally unconnected reason, may turn round and sue him because he has given a much-needed drug during her pregnancy. Where does he turn for advice? He will find little help in general medical journals, which seem more concerned with unconfirmed possibilities, or in review articles which tend to condemn drugs out of context. The drug companies are inclined to say a drug is contra-indicated for medico-legal reasons, without actual evidence. The Committee on Safety of Medicines will comment that their 'contra-indications' merely mean that there are points against the use of certain drugs, rather than that they shouldn't be prescribed. There is little time to consult these sources when there is a pregnant patient waiting for her prescription for drugs which will in fact protect her baby from harm.

Specialist volumes on teratogenesis due to drugs seem to provide little help with everyday clinical practice. Some are based on animal work of limited relevance to human therapeutics; others list every possible association between drugs and congenital abnormalities in the medical literature for reference purposes. Perhaps the most confusing are large scale epidemiological surveys, which reveal hundreds of possible low-level associations, and do not indicate the few that might reflect causal associations of practical clinical meaning. Epidemiologists tend to react along the lines that if we will only wait for ten years, all the answers will be available!

All these problems were emphasised at a meeting on human

teratogenesis held by the Institute of Obstetrics and Gynaecology on 30 May 1980. The speakers were concerned about the very real need of the clinician for guidance through the jungle of pseudo-science and vested interests which befog this field. They are all among the contributors to this book, supporting the view that what is needed is a volume by clinicians — albeit those with specialised knowledge — for clinicians, orientated to the practical needs of treating antenatal and puerperal women.

We started with the principle that information on specific agents, wherever possible, should be based on hard evidence. With such an approach there are inevitably lacunae which can only be filled if the reader is primed with some understanding of the principles of drug-associated teratogenesis and the evaluation of sources of information on these phenomena. It is hoped that the content of the first section, which is concerned with these matters, will provide a critical basis, enabling the reader to use the information on specific therapeutic agents in the second section to the benefit of pregnant patients and their babies. Family practitioners, obstetricians in training and in practice, nurses and midwives, and pharmacists are all concerned in the processes by which antenatal women are given drug treatment and we trust that they will find positive guidance, not just a catalogue of agents about whose use they should be cautious. 'Caution is advised . . .' is one of the most irritating warnings in the reference books on this subject. How can one be cautious about a drug one has to use, without knowing what to be cautious about? We hope that with the drugs dealt with here, sufficient information has been given to indicate the nature of any caution required.

I am grateful to the authors for their patient acceptance of editorial guidance; to Mrs Sylvia Hull of Churchill Livingstone for her encouragement and advice and to Miss Nancy Philcox, Miss Hazel Dixon and Mrs Anne Jones for typing and retyping manuscripts and to publishers who gave permission for reproduction of figures.

London, 1983 D.F.H.

# Contributors

---

**P. J. Bolton,** MB, BS(London), MRCOG.
Consultant in Obstetrics and Gynaecology, Harold Wood Hospital, Essex. Formerly Senior Registrar in Obstetrics and Gynaecology, Hammersmith Hospital, London.

**Patricia A. Crowley,** MB, BCh, DCH, MRCOG, MRCPI.
Registrar, National Maternity Hospital, Dublin. Formerly Glaxo Perinatal Research Fellow, Institute of Obstetrics and Gynaecology, Hammersmith Hospital, London.

**D. F. Hawkins,** PhD, DSc, MB, BS(London); MD(Mass); FRCOG, FACOG.
Professor of Obstetric Therapeutics, Institute of Obstetrics and Gynaecology; Consultant Obstetrician and Gynaecologist, Hammersmith Hospital, London.

**E. L. Hurden,** MSc, PhD.
Clinical Research Associate, Warner Lambert (UK) Ltd, Usk Road, Pontypool, Gwent, Wales. Formerly Research Fellow, Institute of Obstetrics and Gynaecology, Queen Charlotte's Hospital for Women, London.

**R. F. Lamont,** BSc, MB, ChB.
Research Fellow, Institute of Obstetrics and Gynaecology, Hammersmith Hospital, London.

**P. J. Lewis,** MD, MRCP.
Senior Lecturer in Clinical Pharmacology, Royal Postgraduate Medical School; Honorary Consultant Physician, Hammersmith Hospital, London.

**Penelope G. Palmer,** MB, ChB(Otago), FRACP.
Research Fellow, Institute of Child Health, Hammersmith Hospital, London.

**Felicity Reynolds,** MD(London), FFARCS.
Senior Lecturer (Anaesthetics), St Thomas' Hospital Medical School, London.

**Rajinder K. Sidhu,** MB, BS(Punjab), MRCOG.
Lecturer in Obstetrics and Gynaecology, St Thomas' Hospital Medical School, London. Formerly Senior Registrar in Obstetrics and Gynaecology, Hammersmith Hospital, London.

**R. W. Smithells,** MB, BS, FRCP, FRCP Ed., DCH.
Professor of Paediatrics, University of Leeds.

# Contents

# Section one

# 1

*Felicity Reynolds*

# Placental transfer of drugs

The ill effects on the fetus of dread diseases such as syphilis, and of hair raising or non-existent obstetrics have dwindled as both medicine and social conditions have improved. At the same time, if only because they too are potentially remediable, the effects that drugs may have on the baby, once so insignificant, have become relatively more important.

Drugs may affect a fetus either directly, after passage across the placenta, or indirectly, because they alter maternal physiology. Direct effects may be either pharmacological or, if the drug is given at the crucial stage of embryological development, teratogenic. In either case fetal effects are likely to be dose related—this is now fairly well established for teratogenic effects.

Certain drugs are predictably teratogenic. The rapidly dividing fetal cells are likely to be sensitive to agents which affect cell division, enzymes, and protein and DNA synthesis. Thus cytotoxic drugs, the alkylating agents and antimetabolites (Scott 1977) and antibiotics other than penicillin are all potential teratogens. Phenobarbitone given in the sort of doses commonly employed for sedation appears quite innocuous, but given in much larger anticonvulsant doses, in which it may affect folate metabolism, it would appear to carry a teratogenic risk similar to that of phenytoin (Hanson et al 1976). The teratogenic potential of an individual drug in a particular species is disappointingly unpredictable. Many drugs that may become teratogenic when given in large doses to susceptible animal species appear innocuous when used in smaller doses in human pregnancy. Many carcinogenic and mutagenic compounds that might be supposed to be teratogens, act via reactive intermediary products, which are usually highly electrophilic. Such reactive metabolites are likely to be too unstable and non-diffusible to reach the fetus from the maternal circulation. The teratogenic potential of the parent compound therefore depends upon the ability of the fetus to carry out the appropriate metabolic processes. The necessary enzyme systems are present to a small extent in human fetal liver and less so in the placenta, though absent in many experimental animals (Nau and Neubert 1978). Unfortunately, even such pharmacokinetic differences cannot explain much of the interspecies variation in susceptibility to teratogens (Scott et al 1978).

Nevertheless it is safe to say that within one individual or strain, the size of the dose received by the fetus of a single drug or class of compounds plays an important role in teratogenesis. A consideration of placental transfer of drugs and the factors influencing fetal dose, therefore, makes a useful starting point in the study of drug teratogenesis.

*Historically*, concern that drugs given to a pregnant woman might adversely affect the fetus via the placenta was slow to develop. When ether was in its infancy as an anaesthetic, Professor Channing at Harvard pronounced that it did not cross the placenta, since when it was given before delivery he could not detect its smell in the cut ends of the umbilical cord (Caton 1977). The idea became quite widely held that the placenta presented a barrier to drugs. This was odd as its role in the transfer of food and respiratory gases was remarkably well understood by the nineteenth century. John Snow, the father of British anaesthesia, reported in 1853 that he could detect ether in the breath of babies born to mothers who had received it. This was surely a more sensitive assay technique in view of the greater surface area for the generation of smell possessed by the lung than the cut ends of the cord. Moreover, Snow suspected that these neonates were also less active than normal. Widespread concern was slow to arise, because in those days statistics were generally concerned with mortality rather than morbidity, and a successful obstetric outcome was one which resulted in a live mother and a live baby. The development of the Apgar score helped to delineate neonates who suffered immediate depressant effects of drugs, and more recently neurobehavioural assessment scores (Brazelton 1961, 1973, Brackbill et al 1974) have proved much more sensitive detectors of long term neonatal drug effects.

The part that drugs have to play in teratogenesis has proved much more elusive to gatherers of statistics. An explosion in the development of sensitive and specific assay techniques over the past quarter of a century has resulted in a wealth of information concerning placental transfer of drugs, though there are many pitfalls in the interpretation of such data.

## The placental membrane

The human placenta is villous, the villi becoming progressively more branched and so increasing placental surface area as gestation progresses. Initially the chorion possesses two ectodermal layers; the cytotrophoblast, an inner layer of individual cells, and the syncytiotrophoblast, the outer layer. As the surface area of the placenta grows the cytotrophoblast cells cease to form a continuous layer, but preserve the ability to divide for repair of the syncytiotrophoblast. The fetal capillaries are contained in the mesodermal villous cores, and in late gestation come to lie directly beneath thin areas of syncytiotrophoblast, forming vasculosyncytial membranes, areas specialised for rapid diffusion rather than for active metabolic processes. At term, the human placenta is haemomonochorial, a single layer of fetal chorionic tissue separating maternal blood from fetal capillary endothelium.

Thus the surface area available for maternal-fetal exchange increases with gestation, while the membrane becomes progressively thinner. The significance of the syncytial nature of the surface layer lies in the absence of intercellular clefts. Consequently the lipid cell membrane is continuous.

## Placental transfer

Although mechanisms are present for the active transport across the placenta of certain essential substances such as amino acids, drug transfer is in the main by passive diffusion. The same rules govern diffusion here as in other lipid membranes such as the blood-brain barrier, the gastrointestinal tract and the renal tubules. Thus water soluble non-ionised particles diffuse readily across the placenta only with a molecular weight less than 100, while for lipid soluble molecules the maximum size is 600 to 1000. Large water soluble molecules and ions pass only very slowly across lipid membranes.

### *Chemical properties of drugs*

The molecular weights of drugs usually lie in the lower hundreds. All such drugs cross the placenta to some extent. Lipid soluble drugs cross with ease, while water soluble ones pass through only slowly. As a rule of thumb, we can say that drugs which are active when taken by mouth will cross the placenta readily, while those which have to be injected will pass slowly across and are unlikely to reach active concentrations within the fetus, except in unusual circumstances. The distinction between orally effective and ineffective drugs is exemplified by the anticoagulants. Orally effective warfarin can not only occasionally cause fetal bleeding but is also an established teratogen in early pregnancy; heparin, a large, ionised, water soluble mucopolysaccharide of molecular weight 20 000 to 40 000 is relatively safe in pregnancy.

Compounds which are highly ionised, for example quaternary ammonium compounds and penicillin, are always lipid insoluble, and cross the placenta only slowly. Many drugs such as aspirin and barbiturates are weak acids; others, such as antiemetics, tranquillisers and narcotics, are weak bases. By definition these are partially ionised; they cross the placenta in the non-ionised form at a rate dependent upon their lipid solubility. Some drugs used for their central nervous system effects, such as inhalational anaesthetics, ethanol and paracetamol, are non-polar. These are freely lipid soluble and diffusible.

**Factors influencing fetal-maternal concentration ratios**

Many studies purporting to measure placental transfer rate of drugs simply report sundry fetal and maternal blood or plasma concentrations, assayed at intervals following a dose of drug. It is a fallacy to assume that fetal-maternal ratios are a measure of drug permeability. Rate of transfer is not the only influence on this ratio, which is also dependent upon site of sampling of fetal and maternal blood, fetal tissue uptake, and the relative affinities of fetal and maternal blood for the drug.

*Sampling sites*

Maternal blood is commonly sampled from a brachial vein. In view of the different kinetics of fetal blood and maternal forearm blood, the latter is not comparable, in terms of drug concentration, to the uterine vein. Maternal arterial blood samples are more homogeneous, though less ethical. Umbilical vein blood is often sampled though this in no way reflects fetal tissue levels, being directly downstream of the placenta. Fetal arterial blood is not homogeneous, though sampling from the umbilical artery *and* vein can indicate the direction of placental transfer. These strictures about sampling sites apply particularly in a rapidly changing experimental situation, but matter less with chronic drug administration.

*Rate of placental transfer*

This is a term open to various interpretations: 1. rate of movement across the membrane, that is, distance/time; 2. rate of drug transfer, mass/time; or 3. time taken to get from one side to the other. Some workers even imply that fetal-maternal ratios denote *rate* of transfer. From the point of view of fetal dose the second concept (2.) is the important one.

The factors influencing rate of transfer are (a) *placental*: the area and thickness of the membrane and the blood flow on either side; and (b) *drug properties*: diffusible concentration gradient and lipid solubility. Both the area available for maternal-fetal exchange and placental perfusion tend to increase with fetal growth. Both are capable of increasing at high altitude, and may be summarily reduced in, for example, placental infarction or abruption. Theoretical alterations in drug transfer in such circumstances are probably the least of the baby's problems. The placental membrane is thicker in early pregnancy, and this is often supposed to reduce placental drug transfer. True, the time taken to get from one side to the other may be longer and this delays transfer, but it does not necessarily reduce the dose received by the fetus. In the same way, slowing conduction in the atrio-ventricular bundle may retard ventricular contraction but it does not normally reduce ventricular rate. Kanto and Erkkola (1974) attributed a higher fetal-maternal serum ratio for diazepam at term than in early pregnancy to increased placental size and blood flow, and thinning of the trophoblast layers. For the reasons given above their explanations are unlikely, and any alteration in fetal-maternal ratios is much more readily explained by alteration in relative affinities. Diazepam is about 95 per cent bound to protein in adult plasma and only a small increase in binding in the fetus can explain a fetal-maternal ratio greater than 1. It is probable that fetal protein binding is less in early than in late gestation. Thus physiological alterations in the placenta are relatively unimportant in influencing the size of dose of a drug, in mg/kg, received by the fetus.

Drug factors are much more important. The diffusible concentration gradient denotes the gradient for that fraction of drug which is freely diffusible across a lipid membrane; in other words, that which is neither ionised nor bound to plasma protein. Thus for weak acids and bases a high degree of ionisation and high protein binding in maternal plasma both reduce the effective concentration gradient.

Alterations in absolute drug concentration on either side of the placental membrane also affect this gradient. An intravenous bolus of drug in the mother produces a massive but short-lived gradient for diffusion. A full systemic dose of a lipid soluble drug given by this route will produce more placental transfer than if the same dose is given slowly or intramuscularly, when maternal distribution and elimination more readily keep pace with absorption. This applies to even such readily lipid soluble agents as pethidine (Crawford and Rudofsky 1965) and ampicillin (Hirsch et al 1974).

After such a bolus, maternal plasma concentration falls rapidly because tissue uptake is more extensive in mother than fetus, and the gradient may be reversed (see Figure 1.1). This reverse gradient is never large, and transfer from fetus to mother is likely therefore

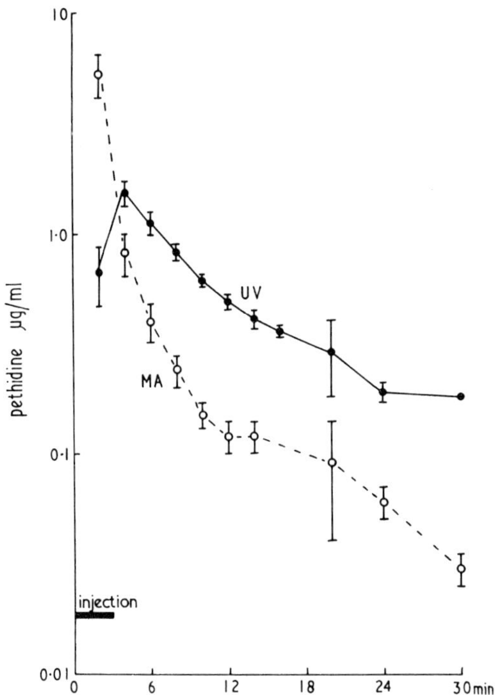


**Figure 1.1** Pethidine concentrations in a maternal artery (MA) and the umbilical vein (UV) in eleven ewes and their lambs following 1.5 mg/kg given intravenously to the mother. (Means ± s.e.) Data from Shier et al 1973, by kind permission of the authors.

to be slower. Fetal elimination is always slower than maternal, and the fetus depends upon placental transfer to eliminate foreign substances. Thus inhalational anaesthetics such as nitrous oxide are rapidly exhaled by the mother, but no such route is available to the fetus *in utero*. Non-volatile lipid soluble drugs must be broken down to hydrophilic metabolites for renal excretion, and the ability of the fetal liver to form water-soluble metabolites such as conjugates is limited (Sanner and Woods 1965, O'Donoghue 1971, Mandelli et al 1975). Indeed this is appropriate, as hydrophilic compounds pass with difficulty across the placenta and so tend to become trapped in the fetal environment. Once fetal kidney function has developed, such compounds may be excreted into the amniotic fluid, only to be drunk by the fetus. Chloramphenicol, an antibiotic which is inactivated by conjugation, is toxic to the neonate, in whom it accumulates unchanged. To the mature fetus, who can eliminate it via the placenta, it is no more toxic than to the adult, though it might of course be teratogenic in early gestation.

A similar story may be told of the local anaesthetic mepivacaine. Sinclair and his colleagues (1965) reported four cases of accidental injection of mepivacaine into the baby's head during attempted caudal block. In each there was fetal bradycardia but the baby was delivered alive within a short period. The first two babies, after convulsing, later died, but the next two survived after exchange transfusion. Could they but have remained *in utero*, nature's own exchange transfusion might well have saved them.

### *Lipid solubility*

There is no such thing in life as absolute impermeability. While it is true that only lipophilic drugs cross the placenta with ease, even totally lipid insoluble drugs do cross, albeit to a small extent.

The placental transfer of the weak base pethidine, by no means the most lipid soluble of the narcotic analgesics, has been widely studied because of its extensive use in labour. Figure 1.1 shows that, if given intravenously to ewes, in whom the placenta is thicker than in the human, within a minute of the end of the injection pethidine concentration in the umbilical vein actually exceeds that in the maternal artery. Thereafter there is probably a biphasic decline in both ewe and lamb, the rate of elimination appearing slightly faster in maternal than in fetal plasma over the short period of the study. It is clear from these data that the clinical importance of any diffusion barrier can be totally discounted.

With barbiturates, rate of transfer can be shown to vary with lipid solubility. The highly lipid soluble anaesthetic induction agent thiopentone, a weak acid which comes into equilibrium across the blood-brain barrier in a single circulation, probably does the same across the placenta. It has a large volume of distribution, so fetal tissue uptake may be prolonged (Finster et al 1972). At the other end of the scale phenobarbitone, also a weak acid but much less lipophilic, crosses the placenta more slowly (Cassano et al 1967) just as it does the blood-brain barrier.

### *Lipid insolubility and the amniotic fluid*

The quaternary ammonium compounds are examples of wholly ionised drugs which are therefore totally hydrophilic. Such are the neuromuscular blocking drugs, much used in clinical anaesthesia and clearly without effect on the neonate when given to the mother before delivery. Sensitive assay techniques can detect these agents in the deceptive umbilical venous blood (Thomas et al 1969, Kivalo and Saarikoski 1972, Booth et al 1977) but effective concentrations

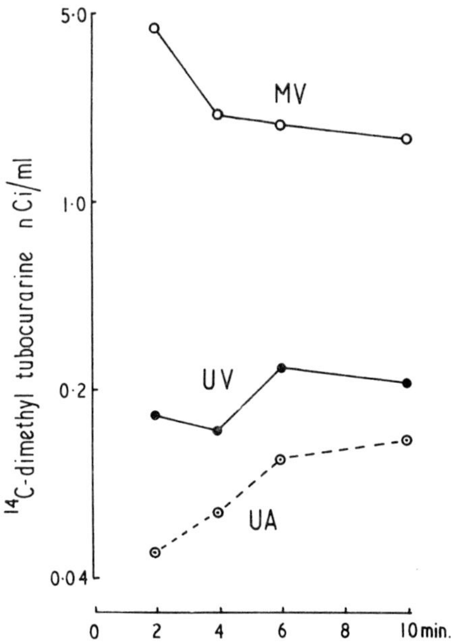


**Figure 1.2** Placental transfer of dimethyl-tubocurarine following a tracer dose of $^{14}$C-labelled compound in 18 patients undergoing caesarean section. MV = maternal vein, UV = umbilical vein, UA = umbilical artery. Data from Kivalo and Saarikoski 1976, by kind permission of the authors.

cannot be demonstrated in the baby when normal doses are given to the mother during clinical anaesthesia (Figure 1.2).

The contrast between Figures 1.1 and 1.2 is clear, and justifies the statement that there is indeed a placental barrier to lipid insoluble foreign compounds. Equilibrium between fetal and maternal plasma is unlikely ever to be achieved for these and other lipid insoluble substances, which tend to accumulate in amniotic fluid once fetal renal function has developed.

Young (1953) gave hexamethonium, the quaternary ammonium ganglion blocker, half-hourly intravenously to does near term and measured its concentration in maternal and fetal plasma and amniotic fluid at varying periods up to twelve hours. Plasma concentrations remained fairly steady, with fetal-maternal ratios about 0.3, but amniotic fluid concentration rose to exceed both, and fell only slowly after stopping administration. Little hexamethonium was measured in the amniotic sacs of those fetuses whose cords had been tied before maternal administration, showing the source was fetal rather than maternal.

It has been shown that lipid insoluble foreign substances in amniotic fluid can come from fetal urine (Basso et al 1977). After a maternal bolus injection in sheep and humans the concentration of the osmotic diuretic mannitol in fetal plasma was low. Amniotic fluid concentration rose to exceed that in maternal and fetal plasma, except in the presence of a dead fetus, or when fetal lamb's urine was voided to the exterior.

Similarly, penicillins, especially benzylpenicillin, have been shown to accumulate in amniotic fluid in late gestation (Wasz–Hockert et al 1970), except when the fetus is dead (Bray et al 1966). Thus hydrophilic compounds tend to accumulate in amniotic fluid because of good renal excretion but poor diffusibility. Penicillins can therefore be used to prevent intra-uterine infection, but only if fetal renal function is good. One can argue that lipid insoluble substances accumulating in the amniotic fluid are unlikely to have any adverse effect upon the fetus. Though he may drink his bathwater such drugs will not be absorbed from his intestine. On the other hand, hexamethonium, which was once given to treat hypertension in pregnancy, could give rise to fetal paralytic ileus. This is hardly surprising since its concentration in the intestinal lumen would be high.

The effect of diffusibility on fetal-maternal ratios is further exemplified by the antibiotics. Orally active ampicillin gives rise to higher fetal concentration than benzylpenicillin, both in early pregnancy (Elek et al 1972) and at term (Wasz-Hockert et al 1970), though after oral administration cord concentrations of ampicillin are rarely therapeutic (Blecher et al 1966). Penicillins as a whole are all more hydrophilic and all cross the placenta less readily than the highly diffusible fusidin, tetracyclines (Kirjuschenkov 1978), chloramphenicol and allied drugs (Bass et al 1978). Moreover the embryotoxicity of these more diffusible classes of antibiotics, which act intracellularly by inhibiting protein synthesis, is readily demonstrated experimentally (Kirjuschenkov 1978, Czempiel et al 1978). The complete absence of both pharmacological reactions and dose-related toxicity of penicillin in the adult is reflected in the fetus. This is not only because of slow placental transfer but also because the bactericidal action of penicillins is selectively on the cell walls; mammalian cells do not possess such overcoats.

*Fetal tissue equilibration*

Lipid soluble drugs cross the placenta very rapidly, the most lipid soluble virtually coming into equilibrium in a single circulation, but they tend to be taken up and concentrated in tissues. Thus full saturation and final equilibration are delayed. Therefore the longer a lipophilic drug is present in maternal plasma, the more it can accumulate in fetal tissues. When a drug is given to the mother, fetal tissues equilibrate much more slowly than maternal, not because they are poorly perfused, but simply because maternal plasma only perfuses the placenta, not the fetal tissues. This may sound obvious, but failure to grasp it has often led investigators to postulate a placental barrier to explain sundry clinical findings and low fetal-maternal ratios.

For example, it is well recognised that it is possible to induce anaesthesia in a woman with a bolus intravenous dose of thiopentone, and then to deliver a baby awake. This is not because of any placental barrier to thiopentone. On the contrary, thiopentone crosses the placenta with ease and probably equilibrates across that membrane, just as it does across the blood-brain barrier. Once across the placenta it encounters further dilution by the rest of the fetal venous return, and a proportion going directly to the fetal liver may be taken up by that organ. The bolus arriving at the fetal brain is a shadow of its former self.

Producing a profound but transient central nervous system effect with a bolus dose is only possible using a very lipid soluble drug, from which recovery occurs by redistribution. Once equilibrated with slower compartments of the body, the concentration is too low for effect. Thus the use of a bolus avoids the need for a full systemic dose of such a drug and gives no chance of equilibration with the slowest compartment of all, the fetus. Mainlining heroin makes use of this bolus effect, and may explain why the babies of addicts who continue to use heroin intravenously sometimes appear to do much better than when the mother has been weaned on to continuous maintenance doses of methadone during pregnancy (E. Tylden, personal communication).

Tissue uptake of drugs by the fetus has been studied in animals rather more than fetal plasma concentrations in early pregnancy because while adequate blood samples are hard to obtain, the small fetus lends itself well to the technique of autoradiography. It is plausible that such localisation of drugs in fetal tissues as has been observed is related to the site of embryotoxicity. Tetracyclines have been shown to be concentrated in the skeleton in the mouse fetus (Ullberg 1973). This chelation of tetracyclines is undoubtedly related to the stunting of growth observed in long bones. Chorpromazine and chloroquine are highly concentrated in the fetal eye (Ullberg 1973, Dencker 1978) and may be associated with retinal damage. It has been suggested that the concentration of diazepam in the heart may be related to the inhibition of reflex control of heart rate (Sereni 1973, Mandelli et al 1975).

*Relative affinities of maternal and fetal plasma*

Differences in affinity of fetal and maternal plasma for drugs is one of the most important factors influencing fetal-maternal ratios of freely permeable drugs, and one which is most frequently overlooked. Differences in affinity are greatest with weak acids and bases, for two reasons. One is that there is a pH gradient across the placenta of about 0.1 of a pH unit. The pH affects the ionisation of weak electrolytes, acids being more ionised at higher pH and bases at low pH. Since only the non-ionised fraction is freely permeable, at equilibrium an acidic compound tends to be more concentrated in the more alkaline maternal medium, while a base is concentrated in the fetus. This phenomenon in general is known as ion trapping. The effect on the relative concentrations of free drug across the placenta is slight, but if fetal pH falls because of impaired placental function the fetal-maternal ratio of a basic drug may rise. This has been shown for local anaesthetics given in labour (Kennedy et al 1979) and despite impaired placental function the fetal dose of a potentially depressant basic drug may actually rise.

The more important influence on fetal-maternal ratios of weak electrolytes is protein binding. The affinity of maternal plasma proteins is higher than fetal for local anaesthetics (Reynolds 1970, Tucker et al 1970, Thomas et al 1976) and phenobarbitone and phenytoin (Ehrnebo et al 1971) but lower for salicylates (Levy et al 1975). The affinity of fetal plasma is higher than maternal for diazepam; fetal-maternal ratios of about 2 are usually measured (Mandelli et al 1975, Erkkola et al 1973). Lower ratios than this have sometimes been recorded in early pregnancy (Kanto and Erkkola 1974). Such a difference, if not simply due to incomplete equilibration after short-term administration, is much more likely caused by the lower affinity of immature plasma proteins than by any reduced placental permeability in early pregnancy. Any barrier to diffusion is biologically impossible with such a lipid soluble drug.

## Conclusion

By far the most important chemical property of a drug which determines the pharmacokinetics of potential embryotoxicity is its lipid solubility. Lipid soluble drugs cross the placenta rapidly and with ease, but as they tend to be taken up in fetal as well as maternal tissues, they are very slowly cumulative in the fetus. Thus the longer the maternal administration of a drug, and the slower its elimination from the maternal environment, the more likely is it that the fetus receives a dose which may be toxic. A hydrophilic drug, on the other hand, is slow to cross the placenta, and although theoretically it may ultimately equilibrate across the placenta in early pregnancy if administration is prolonged, it is limited in its distribution to the extracellular compartment, and by its very nature is unlikely to affect cell growth and division. In later gestation it is likely to be eliminated rapidly in the urine of both fetus and mother, and can become trapped in amniotic fluid and fetal gastro-intestinal tract.

## REFERENCES

Bass R, Schutte I, Nau H 1978 Placental transfer and fetal distribution of thiaphenicol in pregnant rats and humans. In: Neubert D, Merker H-J, Nau H, Langman J (editors) Role of pharmacokinetics in prenatal and perinatal toxicology. Georg Thieme, Stuttgart, pp 507–518

Basso A, Fernandez A, Althabe O, Sabini G, Piriz H, Belitzky R 1977 Passage of mannitol from mother to amniotic fluid and fetus. Obstetrics and Gynecology 49: 628–631

Blecher T E, Edgar W M, Melville H A H, Peel K R 1966 Transplacental passage of ampicillin. British Medical Journal i: 137–139

Booth P N, Watson M J, McLeod K 1977 Pancuronium and the placental barrier. Anaesthesia 32: 320–323

Brackbill Y, Kane J, Manniello R L, Abramson D 1974 Obstetric premedication and infant outcome. American Journal of Obstetrics and Gynecology 118: 377–384

Bray R E, Boe R W, Johnson W L 1966. Transfer of ampicillin into fetus and amniotic fluid from maternal plasma in late pregnancy. American Journal of Obstetrics and Gynecology 96: 938–942

Brazelton T B 1961 Psychophysiological reactions in the neonate. II Effect of maternal medication on the neonate and his behaviour. Journal of Pediatrics 58: 513–518

Brazelton T B 1973 Assessment of the infant at risk. Clinical Obstetrics and Gynecology 16: 361–375

Cassano G B, Ghetti B, Gliozzi E, Hansson E 1967 Autoradiographic distribution study of 'short-acting' and 'long-acting' barbiturates: $^{35}$S-thiopentone and $^{14}$C-phenobarbitone. British Journal of Anaesthesia 39: 11–20

Caton D 1977 Obstetric anesthesia and concepts of placental transport. A historical review of the nineteenth century. Anesthesiology 46: 132–137

Crawford J S, Rudofsky S 1965 The placental transmission of pethidine. British Journal of Anaesthesia 37: 929–933

Czempiel W, Ulbrich B, Bass R 1978 The effects of chloramphenicol and its analogues on 55S, 70S, and 80S ribosomes: the implication to their embryotoxic mode of action. In: Neubert D, Merker H-J, Nau H, Langman J (editors) Role of pharmacokinetics in prenatal and perinatal toxicology. Georg Thieme, Stuttgart, pp 527–534

Dencker L 1978 Localization of diffusible substances in the embryo. In: Neubert D, Merker H-J, Nau H, Langman J (editors) Role of pharmacokinetics in prenatal and perinatal toxicology. Georg Thieme, Stuttgart, pp 535–544

Ehrnebo M, Agurell S, Jalling B, Boreus L O 1971 Age differences in drug binding by plasma proteins; studies on human foetuses, neonates and adults. European Journal of Clinical Pharmacology 3: 189–193

Elek E, Ivan E, Arr M 1972 Passage of penicillins from mother to foetus in humans. International Journal of Clinical Pharmacology and Therapeutic Toxicology 6: 223–225

Erkkola R, Kangas L, Pekkerinen A 1973 The transfer of diazepam across the placenta during labour. Acta obstetricia et gynecologica Scandinavica 52: 167–170

Finster M, Morishima H O, Mark L C, Perel J M, Dayton P G, James L S 1972 Tissue thiopental concentrations in the fetus and newborn. Anethesiology 36: 155–158

Hanson J W, Myrianthopoulos N C, Harvey M A S, Smith D W 1976 Risks to the offspring of women treated with hydantoin anticonvulsants with emphasis on the fetal hydantoin syndrome. Journal of Pediatrics 89: 662–668

Hirsch H A, Dreher E, Schmid E 1974 Transfer of ampicillin to the fetus and amniotic fluid during continuous infusion (steady state) and by repeated single intravenous injections to the mother. Infection 2: 207–212

Kanto J, Erkkola R 1974 The feto-maternal distribution of diazepam in early human pregnancy. Annales chirurgiae et gynaecologiae 63: 489–491

Kennedy R L, Erenberg A, Robillard J E, Merkow A, Turner T 1979 Effects of changes in maternal-fetal pH on the transplacental equilibrium of bupivacaine. Anesthesiology 51: 50–54

Kirjuschenkov A P 1978 Embryotoxicity of antibiotics. In: Neubert D, Merker H-J, Nau H, Langman J (editors) Role of pharmacokinetics in prenatal and perinatal toxicology. Georg Thieme, Stuttgart, pp 591–593

Kivalo I, Saarikoski S 1972 Placental transmission and foetal uptake of $^{14}$C-dimethyltubocurarine. British Journal of Anaesthesia 44: 557–561

Kivalo I, Saarikoski S 1976 Placental transfer of $^{14}$C-dimethyltubocurarine during caesarian section. British Journal of Anaesthesia 48: 239–242

Levy G, Procknal J A, Garrettson L K 1975 Distribution of salicylate between neonatal and maternal serum at diffusion equilibrium. Clinical Pharmacology and Therapeutics 18: 210–214

Mandelli M, Morselli P L, Nordio S, Pardi G, Principi N, Sereni F, ıgnoni G 1975 Placental transfer of diazepam and its disposition in the newborn. Clinical Pharmacology and Therapeutics 17: 564–572

Nau H, Neubert D 1978 Development of drug-metabolizing mono-oxygenase systems in various mammalian species including man. Its significance for transplacental toxicity. In: Neubert D, Merker H-J, Nau H, Langman J (editors) Role of pharmacokinetics in prenatal and perinatal toxicology. Georg Thieme, Stuttgart, pp 13–44

O'Donoghue S E F 1971 Distribution of pethidine and chlorpromazine in maternal, foetal and neonatal biological fluids. Nature 229: 124

Reynolds F 1970 Systemic toxicity of local analgesic drugs with special reference to bupivacaine. M D Thesis, University of London

Sanner J H, Woods L A 1965 Comparative distribution of tritium-labelled dihydromorphine between maternal and fetal rats. Journal of Pharmacology and Experimental Therapeutics 148: 176–184

Scott J R 1977 Fetal growth retardation associated with maternal administration of immunosuppressive drugs. American Journal of Obstetrics and Gynecology 128: 668–676

Scott W J, Wilson J G, Ritter E J, Fradkin R 1978 Further studies on distribution of teratogenic drugs in pregnant rats and rhesus monkeys. In: Neubert D, Merker H-J, Nau H, Langman J (editors) Role of pharmacokinetics in prenatal and perinatal toxicology. Georg Thieme, Stuttgart, pp 499–505

Sereni F 1973 The need for further data. In: Symposium: drugs and the unborn child. Clinical Pharmacology and Therapeutics 14: 662–665

Shier R W, Sprague A D, Dilts P V 1973 Placental transfer of meperidine HCl. Part II. American Journal of Obstetrics and Gynecology 115: 556–559

Sinclair J C, Fox H A, Lentz J F, Fuld G L, Murphy J 1965 Intoxication of the fetus by a local anesthetic. New England Journal of Medicine 273: 1173–1177

Thomas J, Climie C R, Mather L E 1969 The placental transfer of alcuronium. British Journal of Anaesthesia 41: 297–302

Thomas J, Long G, Moore G, Morgan D 1976 Plasma protein binding and placental transfer of bupivacaine. Clinical Pharmacology and Therapeutics 19: 426–434

Tucker G T, Boyes R N, Bridenbaugh P O and Moore D C 1970 Binding of anilide-type local anesthetics in human plasma:II. Implications in vivo, with special reference to transplacental distribution. Anesthesiology 33: 304–314

Ullberg S 1973 Autoradiography in fetal pharmacology. In: Borius L (editor) Fetal pharmacology. Raven Press, New York, pp 55–69

Wasz-Hockert O, Nummi S, Vuopala S, Jarvinen P A 1970 Transplacental passage of azidocillin, ampicillin and penicillin G during early and late pregnancy. Scandinavian Journal of Infectious Diseases 2: 125–130

Young M 1953 The placental transfer of hexamethorium bromide and the origin of amniotic fluid in the rabbit. Journal of Physiology 122: 93–101

*Peter J. Lewis*

# Animal tests for teratogenicity, their relevance to clinical practice

Clinicians looking after pregnant women have every right to complain about the present situation on drugs used in early pregnancy. Twenty years after the thalidomide disaster teratologists are still not able to provide them with answers to the most important frequently asked questions on drugs and early pregnancy: 1. Is this drug safe in early pregnancy? 2. Is this drug, which my patient took in early pregnancy, responsible for the child's birth defect?

Unfortunately just because a question is simple and straightforward there is no guarantee that the answer will be similarly and straightforward! In the present state of knowledge, neither of these fundamental questions can be answered with much certainty, largely because animal tests of teratogenicity are simply not accurate predictors of teratogenic effects in man.

## Teratogenicity tests in animals

At present new drugs for human use are subjected to animal tests of teratogenicity and in Western countries these are all variants of the Food and Drug Administration guidelines first issued in 1966 (Wilson 1979). Essentially, at least two animal species are used for these tests and the drugs are administered at 2 or 3 dose levels. No drug authorities require teratological testing in primates and the usual species used are rats and rabbits. Unfortunately these animal tests are very poor predictors of safety in human pregnancy.

### *False negative animal tests*

Thalidomide is a drug in a class apart as a human teratogen. So far as is known, no similar substance exists with as great a teratogenic effect in man, where even a single tablet of the drug taken at a critical period during development can produce teratogenic effects. Despite this, it is difficult to show that thalidomide is a teratogen in animal tests. Schardein (1975) writes 'In approximately 10 strains of rats, 15 strains of mice, 11 breeds of rabbit, 2 breeds of dogs, 3 strains of hamsters, 8 species of primates and in such other varied species as cats, armadillos, guinea-pigs, swine and ferrets in which thalidomide has been tested, teratogenic effects have been induced only occasionally.' Phocomelia, the characteristic defect in man, has been produced in seven species of primate, but in all these species higher doses of drugs are necessary to produce the deformity than in man.

Since few other drugs are accepted as teratogens in man, even to the extent of causing small increases in common abnormalities, it is difficult to give further examples of false negative tests in animals.

*False positive animal tests*

Several drugs cause malformation in laboratory animals but not in man. These examples of incongruence have always been attacked because evidence of complete safety of drugs in man is difficult to accept. Aspirin, caffeine and acetazolamide are all substances which have been or are in common use in pregnant women and none has been associated with any characteristic malformation in humans (Layton 1974). Aspirin is a teratogen in the rat, mouse, monkey, guinea-pig, cat and dog (Robertson et al 1979). The active teratogenic metabolite in rats, salicyclic acid, is also produced by metabolism in humans.

In general, small laboratory animals are more susceptible to teratogens than are higher primates. Of the approximately 2000 chemical compounds which have been tested for teratogenicity in laboratory animals about a third can be classified as teratogens in one species or another (Schardein 1975). The relative paucity of substances which are accepted as having a teratogenic effect in man suggests that small laboratory animals are also much more susceptible to teratogenic effects than is man.

*Why are animal tests inaccurate?*

The rationale for believing that teratogenicity in one species will accurately predict teratogenicity in another species is rather obscure. Consider a model situation. If we take any other species than man, say the cat, and attempt to predict teratogenicity in this species by testing in other species such as the rat and the rabbit, then we can easily demonstrate the inutility of the test procedure. It is evident that teratogenicity tests in one species do not predict teratogenicity in another unless the relationship is very close.

Indeed, it would be surprising if there was congruence in view of what is known of the mechanisms of teratogenicity. Biotransformation in the fetus is a prerequisite for many teratogenic effects and differences in biotransformation patterns in different species and even in different strains of the same species are very profound. Besides biotransformation in the fetus itself, the placenta and mother are other sites of metabolism which have potentially different activities from one species to another. Furthermore, different individuals of the same species can differ quite profoundly in their biotransformation patterns for the same drug (Balke et al 1979, Shum et al 1979). For example, it has recently been shown that there is a multiplicity of different cycochrome p-450 enzymes in the liver (Ryan et al 1979). *In vitro* measurement of various p-450 components in human liver has shown an astonishing range of inter-individual differences and this presumably accounts for the different pattern of metabolites which different individuals produce when dosed with the same drug. Metabolic differences between species and between individuals of the same species are likely to be major determinants of whether a drug is teratogenic for one individual but not for another.

Pharmacokinetic differences have been appreciated as potential confounding factors in teratogenicity testing for some time (Layton 1974). The placentas of different animals are so different that the speed and amount of drug transfer to the fetus differs from species to species, although this factor is probably not as important as the differences in biotransformation.

Even if the drug were to reach the fetus or embryo of different species at the same concentration and be transferred to a similar metabolite in the same way, then variations might still occur in the individual's response to the potential teratogen (Bustamante and Stumpff 1978). For all these various reasons, the potential lack of correlation between species as far as teratogenicity is concerned is not difficult to understand.

## Implications

The poor predictive value of animal teratogenicity tests has been apparent for years. One may ask then why these tests are still done and still required by drug regulatory authorities, as they are obviously not efficacious for the purpose for which they are apparently performed. This may be a slightly naive view since, although the tests are virtually useless scientifically, we have nothing to replace them with and they do fulfil at least one function: to provide some defence against public allegations of neglect of adequate drug testing. In other words, something is being done, although it is not the right thing. Furthermore, animal teratogenicity tests cost a good deal of money and provide employment for a large section of the scientific community. Lack of efficacy seems almost irrelevant in assessing such a vested interest. These tests will continue to be required for the foreseeable future.

*Better tests*

It seems likely that the present stalemate on drugs for use in pregnancy will continue for some time yet. There is simply no way in which, on present knowledge, predictions of safety or danger can be made. At present, the safety of a drug in pregnancy can only be assessed until a reasonable number of pregnant women have been fortuitously exposed to it on a number of occasions.

The plain fact is that even if a horrendous totalitarian regime were able to perform teratogenicity tests on the human species itself using some subjugate 'inferior race' it seems likely that the test procedure would still fall short of the totally satisfactory. The interaction of teratogen and genetic make up of the mother and fetus is so complex that, at least for minor teratogens, huge numbers of unfortunate experimental subjects would be necessary in order to produce any convincing results.

Other approaches such as embryo culture (Shepard and Robkin 1976) and mutagenicity tests are even further removed from the clinical situation and are incapable of being validated or accepted.

## Conclusions

In the absence of useful tests of teratogenicity clinicians have to accept the responsibility for drug exposures in early pregnancy. The ideal of all prescribing practice, that drugs are only used for proper indications and when potential benefit is likely to outweigh potential harm, must be rigorously applied in pregnant women. Unfortunately the reality in clinical practice often falls short of this standard. If clinicians were more aware of the shortcomings of animal teratogenicity testing they might take this responsibility more seriously.

## REFERENCES

Balke D A, Martz F, Martz A G, Gordon G B, Mellits E D 1979 Fetal tissues from various strains of induced mice metabolise benzo(a)pyrene to mutagenic metabolites. Teratology 20: 377–382

Bustamante S A, Stumpff I C 1978 Fetal hydantoin syndrome in triplets. American Journal of Diseases of Children 132: 978–979

Layton W M 1974 An analysis of teratogenic testing procedures. In: Janerich D T, Skalko R G, Porter I H (editors) Congenital defects. Academic Press, New York, pp 205–217

Robertson R T, Henry L A, Bokelman D L 1979 Aspirin: teratogenic evaluation in the dog. Teratology 20: 313–320

Ryan D E, Thomas P E, Korzeniowski D, Levin W 1979 Separation and characterization of highly purified forms of liver microsomal cytochrome p-450 from rats treated with polychlorinated biphenyls, phenobarbital, and 3-methylcholanthrene. Journal of Biological Chemistry 254: 1365–1374

Schardein J L 1975 Drugs as teratogens. CRC Press, Cleveland, Ohio

Shepard T H, Robkin M 1976 The use of whole mammalian embryo culture in studies of teratogenesis. In: Tests of teratogenicity in vitro. North Holland, Amsterdam, pp 435–448

Shum S, Jensen N M, Nebert D W 1979 The murine Ah locus: in utero toxicity and teratogenesis associated with genetic differences in benzo(a)pyrene metabolism. Teratology 20: 365–376

Wilson J G 1979 The evolution of teratological testing: Teratology 20: 205–212

# 3

*R. W. Smithells*

# The demonstration of teratogenic effects of drugs in humans

Although it is now 20 years since the teratogenic effects of thalidomide were first reported, public interest in the general topic of teratogenesis has waxed rather than waned. This is partly because of the instinctive fear of having a malformed baby and anxiety to avoid such a tragedy if possible, but largely because of teratogenesis lawsuits, and the extensive and often inaccurate coverage accorded to them by the media. In this paper I have been asked 'to inject some sense and realism' into the subject, to take a careful scientific look at a topic which inevitably arouses emotions. The central question may be put thus: how are we to determine whether a particular drug is causing, or contributing to the causation of, human birth defects?

The problem is complex, and if it is to become understandable certain concepts have to be clarified.

## SOME GENERAL PRINCIPLES

### Teratogenic effects

The first is to define just what is meant by a teratogenic effect. There is a range of phenomena which can be called teratogenic effects (Table 3.1). The damage that can be done to humans in the prenatal period includes spontaneous abortion, the major structural defects which are the subject of most papers on teratogenicity, minor structural defects, prenatal and postnatal growth retardation, develop-

**Table 3.1** The natural spectrum of teratogenic effects

| |
|---|
| Spontaneous abortion |
| Major structural defects |
| Minor structural defects |
| Prenatal growth retardation |
| Postnatal growth retardation |
| Developmental retardation |
| Behaviour disorders |

mental retardation, defects of hearing and vision, and behavioural disorders. If it is accepted that alcohol has teratogenic potential in humans, it can probably produce most of these abnormalities, as can congenital rubella. Teratogenicity is not just the ability to produce congenital structural abnormalities: it is potentially a much wider field.

### Teratogenic agents

A teratogenic agent in its broadest sense could be defined as anything which increases the chances of a baby being born with a structural or functional abnormality. In this context we tend to think of positive agents such as a teratogenic drug, alcohol (which is a drug if you are teetotal. but not if you drink it yourself!), a food additive, an air pollutant; even an Irish dock labourer, because his child is more likely to be born with spina bifida than the child of a middle-class Englishman. The contribution of drugs to human teratogenesis is probably very small, but a more fastidious approach to prescribing in pregnancy might diminish slightly the risk of birth defects.

Teratogenic effects can also be due to negative factors. Omission of rubella vaccination is perhaps a tortuous example, but there is growing evidence that minor deficiencies of one or more vitamins may contribute to the causation of neural tube defects. By making good the deficiency, prevention may be possible (Smithells et al 1981).

When teratogenic effects in humans are being considered, the discussion usually relates to babies born, because the 'incidence' of birth defects is defined in these terms. But many malformed fetuses are aborted spontaneously (Nishimura 1970). Nature has devised a remarkably efficient system for the disposal of an abnormal conceptus. Anything which interferes with that process can be said to have a teratogenic effect, as tending to produce an increased incidence of malformations recognised after 28 weeks. This hypothesis is difficult to test, particularly in regard to antinauseants, because there is continuing support for the curious observation that pregnancy nausea and vomiting are inversely related to the occurrence of spontaneous abortion. This illustrates the sort of interaction that bedevils studies of teratogenesis. The more vomiting there is, the more drugs are given; and the fewer the abortions.

### Specificity

By specificity is meant that the pattern of disturbed growth and development attributable to an agent is clearly recognisable, whether one or several body systems are affected. Thalidomide can affect not only the limbs but practically every organ in the body, and yet produces a highly specific complex of effects. The effects are so characteristic that thalidomide can be incriminated with a high degree of confidence even when there is no documentary evidence that the mother actually took the drug. As an example of non-specificity we may consider hormone pregnancy tests, now withdrawn from sale because of a faint possibility that they may be teratogenic. The total evidence is not very persuasive, partly because the effects described lack specificity. When the literature relating sex hormones to birth defects is studied, we find positive associations reported with spina bifida, anencephaly, congenital heart disease, cleft lip, cleft palate, hypospadias, cataract, limb defects and others, but (with the exception of cardiac lesions) none of these associations turns up more than once (Smithells 1981). One reason for this lies in the design of the investigations, but overall the data do not hang together. This contrasts with thalidomide, where the pattern of abnormalities is coherent in the scientific sense.

### Minor Teratogens and Multifactorial Causation

To say something is teratogenic implies a simple causal relationship. In practice, the cause and effect relationship is seldom as simple as that. An example is shown in Figure 3.1. A is the agent with which we are concerned, B and C are other factors and E is the effect. In Figure 3.1(a) agent A is the cause of effect E and the latter can only be brought about by the exhibition of agent A. Such a one-to-one relationship is rare in real life, although certain genetic examples exist. Anyone who has the genes of chromosome 21 present in triplicate will show the clinical features of Down's syndrome and vice versa. Thalidomide taken at the relevant stage of gestation was, for practical purposes, 100 per cent teratogenic.

In Figure 3.1(b), agent A may be followed by effect E, but the same effect can result from other causes. For example, warfarin given in pregnancy can produce in the human fetus a form of punctate epiphyseal dysplasia which is clinically and radiologically indistinguishable from the same disease occurring in the offspring of women who have not had warfarin. Agent A is *a* cause of E, but not the only cause.

By far the commonest real-life situation is indicated in Figure 3.1(c). Agent A may be followed by effect E, but there are also women who have taken the same drug in the same dose through the same period of pregnancy and have given birth to babies that did not manifest effect E. Anticonvulsants are a clear example. The babies of epileptic mothers who have taken these drugs during preg-

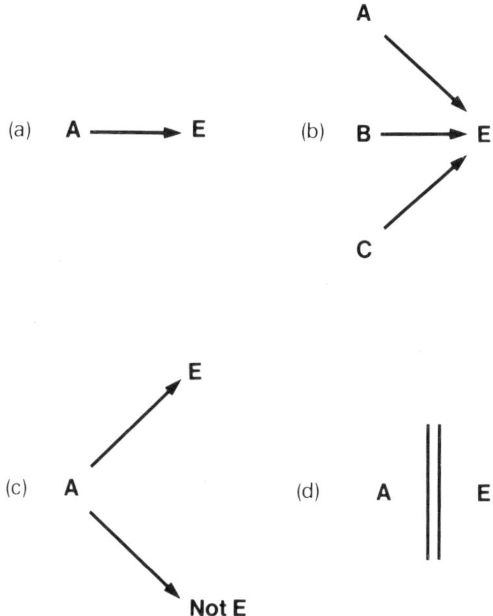


**Figure 3.1** (a) *One to one cause and effect relationship*. A is *the* cause of E. A is invariably preceded by A. (b) *Alternative causation*. A is *a* cause of E. A is invariably followed by E; E is not always preceded by A. (c) *A causes E if other factors are operative*. A causes E sometimes (that is, under some circumstances). Factors other than A determine whether E will follow. (d) *No causal relatioship*. A never causes E. A is never followed by E; E is never preceded by A. (Reproduced by permission of MTP Press Ltd, Lancaster).

nancy have an increased incidence of congenital anomalies, particularly facial clefts and congenital heart disease (Meadow 1979). A specific fetal phenytoin syndrome has also been described. But the great majority of babies born to epileptics under treatment have no congenital defects. Thus, A is *sometimes* followed by E. This is another way of saying that A on its own is not sufficient to cause E, which only results if other genetic or environmental contributory factors co-exist.

Figure 3.1(d) illustrates the situation where A has no causal connection with E, even though some factor common to both may lead to a significant association.

We need to understand the terms 'sufficient cause', 'necessary cause' and 'contributory cause'. Consider pulmonary tuberculosis. The tubercle bacillus is a necessary cause in that tuberculosis cannot occur without it. On the other hand the tubercle bacillus is not a sufficient cause, as a patient can encounter the organism, as evidenced by a positive tuberculin skin test, without developing any clinical disease. Other contributory causes determine whether or not the disease tuberculosis develops. Any combination of necessary and contributory causes which invariably has a predicted effect adds up to sufficient cause. The contributory factors which go to make up a sufficient cause may be quite different in different people.

Hence if a drug is called a minor teratogen, it means that it is not of itself a sufficient cause of birth defect as was thalidomide. It means that the drug will only exert a teratogenic effect on some embryos, and therefore that other contributory factors must be involved. Nearly all congenital malformations in the human are multifactorial in origin. Whether or not an embryo develops normally depends on a balance of influences. On the one side are factors tending to facilitate normal growth and development: on the other are factors tending to frustrate it. If we talk about a drug as a minor teratogen, it is merely one component in the balance and is no more or less a teratogen than any of the other factors. A crude analogy may be drawn with road accidents. These are scarcely ever attributable to a single factor. It is the combination of a tired driver, a wet road, a stray dog, a worn tyre and one drink too many that add up to a road accident. Even the police have changed from specifying the cause of an accident to considering its causes, in the plural.

## DEMONSTRATION OF TERATOGENIC EFFECTS OF DRUGS

### Clinical associations

These might be termed 'inspirations', and the first in the field of human teratogenesis was undoubtedly Gregg's (1941) observation of the link between rubella in pregnancy and cataract in the baby. The insight was not a matter of thinking up a new idea, but of paying attention to what his patients told him. Similarly with thalidomide, Lenz (1961) linked bizarre limb defects with the drug Contergan. Clinical observation at the personal level will probably always be the most fruitful source of ideas about teratogens affecting humans. They will rarely be sufficient to confirm the suspicions they produce or to measure the magnitude of the risk.

### Population Monitoring

Birth defect monitoring was the pastime of the few before 1960, but now consumes considerable resources world-wide. It is tedious, time-consuming and not very fruitful. It has not yet identified a single hitherto unsuspected teratogen, but does provide a mechanism by which suspicions can be aroused. It will continue for a mixture of scientific and political reasons.

**Post-marketing surveillance**

This holds a lot of promise. Even after extensive animal tests we still have no real idea what a drug will do to humans. After clinical trials there comes a day when the drug is marketed. At the present time, once the drug is generally available little further notice seems to be taken, in the hope that all will be well. The concept of deliberately looking for adverse effects, not just teratogenic effects, makes a great deal of sense. Post-marketing surveillance is relatively easy for prescribed drugs, because the prescription (under the National Health Service in Great Britain) can be used to identify patients by whom it has been taken (Inman 1980).

**Epidemiological studies**

These comprise the bulk of the literature on drug teratology in man, and form the main basis on which we must decide whether or not a drug is teratogenic. The design can be either retrospective or prospective. That is, we can either start with a study group of malformed babies and go back into the histories of the mothers, or we can start with a study group of mothers who take a given drug and see how their babies turn out. Ideally there should be some kind of control group with which to make comparisons. A retrospective survey with controls is a 'case control' study; a prospective study, with or without controls, is a 'cohort study'.

*Retrospective studies* may result in pseudo-specificity. Work that starts with a group of children with congenital heart disease and goes back into their histories tells us nothing about whether or not the drug concerned is also associated with limb defects. Another limitation of retrospective studies arises if information about drug intake is sought from the mothers. This is recall bias. The mother of a malformed baby racks her brains for a possible cause for the defect, considering amongst other things the drugs she took during pregnancy. People are more likely to remember prescribed drugs than those they bought over the counter because, at least subconsciously, they feel guilty and are trying to pin the blame on somebody else. The mother who has produced a normal baby will not spend time racking her brains to help other people's research.

*Prospective studies* are limited by the fact that most mothers produce normal babies and very large numbers have to be studied in order to include a meaningful number of abnormal babies. A legitimate prospective study can be done retrospectively by going back to what was recorded in the case notes before it was known whether or not the baby was normal. If the records are completely accurate this can be a good study, but they very rarely are.

Controls are a great problem. A study group can be compared with the population from which they are drawn, provided one takes into account the period of time in which the study was carried out and where the mothers or the babies come from geographically. Alternatively, matched controls can be used. This is epidemiologically respectable, but it is a delusion to believe that if two women are matched for race, age and parity, there are no significant differences between them. If controls are matched by as many as ten relevant characteristics this may be more meaningful, but not much more. Matching can only be for factors which are known to be relevant. There may be very important factors which are not known about. The easiest way to criticise a controlled study in humans is to say that the controls are unacceptable; the criticism can nearly always be substantiated. There is only one way to get round these criticisms.

*Randomised trials*. Suppose we are studying a drug for treating vomiting in pregnancy. The first step is to define the criteria for admission to the study. As appropriate patients present they may be randomly divided into a group that will be given the test drug and a group that will receive nothing or a placebo. The two groups are then likely to be broadly comparable. If we are testing the effect on sickness, in which there is a subjective element, the researcher should be 'blind'. If there is a placebo group, the patients should be 'blind'. If we are testing for teratogenicity, 'blindness' is less important. Interestingly, the first seems to be ethically acceptable, the second not, although precisely the same thing is to be done. Nonetheless, such random allocation is the only way of achieving strict comparability.

At the end of the study a statistically significant association between the drug and a defect may have been detected. Even then, uncertainty remains as whether or not there is any cause and effect relationship (Hill 1965). The stronger the association, the more likely is it to be one of cause and effect. Consistency is also important: if other studies confirm the association, it is more likely to mean causation. The degree of specificity of the teratogenic effect is also important. When dealing with suspected teratogenicity of a drug, the nature of the malformation must be consistent with the stage of pregnancy at which it was taken. Dose-response relationships are not always helpful: with thalidomide a very small dose given at the relevant time could do a great deal of harm. Finally, does the proposed relationship have the overall appearance of validity? Do all the studies, looking at the problem from different angles, fit together in a coherent way, and is the evidence analogous to that in other, well-substantiated situations? These are the sort of useful pointers that provide guides as to whether or not a statistically significant association really means anything in clinical terms.

## SAFETY OF DRUGS IN PREGNANCY

The concept of absolute safety of drugs needs to be demolished. It has been suggested that a particular antinauseant used in pregnancy (Debendox) should have been taken off the market until it could be proved to be safe. In real life it can never be shown that a drug (or anything else) has no teratogenic activity at all, in the sense of never being a contributory factor in anybody under any circumstances. This concept can neither be tested nor proved.

Let us suppose, for example, that some agent doubles the incidence of a condition that has 'natural' incidence of 1 in 10 000 births. If the hypothesis is true, then studying 20 000 pregnant women who have taken the drug and 20 000 who have not may yield respectively two cases and one case of the abnormality. It does not take a statistician to realise that this signifies nothing, and it may need ten times as many pregnant women (almost half a million) to produce a statistically significant result. This would involve such an extensive multicentre study that hundreds of doctors and hospitals have to participate. The participants then each tend to bend the protocol to fit in with their clinical customs and in the end it is difficult to assess the validity of the data. Alternatively, a limited geographical basis may be used, with the trial going on for many years. During this time other things in the environment change, so again the results would not command our confidence. If it were to be suggested that there was something slightly teratogenic in milk, the hypothesis would be virtually untestable.

In practice we have to make up our minds which drugs may reasonably be given to pregnant women. Do we start from a position of presumed guilt or from one of presumed innocence? If the former course is chosen then we cannot give any drugs to pregnant women because we can never prove that they are completely free of teratogenic influence. It therefore seems that we must start from a position of presumed innocence and then take all possible steps to find out if the presumption is correct.

Finally, we must put the matter in perspective by considering the benefit/risk ratio. The problem of prescription in pregnancy cannot be considered from the point of view of only one side of the equation. Drugs are primarily designed to do good, and if a pregnant woman is ill it is in the best interests of her baby and herself that she gets better as quickly as possible. This often means giving her drugs. We can argue about the necessity of giving drugs to prevent vomiting, but there is no argument about the need for treatment of women with meningitis, septicaemia or venereal disease.

What we must try to avoid is medication by the media or prescription by politicians. A public scare about a well-tried drug will lead to wider use of less-tried alternatives. We do not want to be forced to practise the kind of defensive medicine that is primarily designed to avoid litigation. The best decisions for patients are made by well-informed doctors.

## REFERENCES

Gregg M M 1941 Congenital cataract following german measles in the mother. Transactions of the Ophthalmic Society of Australia 3: 35–46

Hill A B 1965 The environment and disease: association and causation. Proceedings of the Royal Society of Medicine 58: 295–300

Inman W H W 1980 The United Kingdom. In: Inman W H W (editor) Monitoring for Drug Safety. MTP Press, Lancaster, pp 9–47

Lenz W 1962 Thalidomide and congenital abnormalities. Lancet i: 45

Meadow S R 1979 Congenital malformations and seizure disorders in offspring of parents with epilepsy. Developmental Medicine and Child Neurology 21: 536–537

Nishimura H 1970 Incidence of malformations in abortions. In: Fraser F C, McKusick V A, Robinson R (editors) Congenital malformations. Excerpta Medica, Amsterdam, pp 275–283

Smithells R W 1981 Oral contraceptives and birth defects. Developmental Medicine and Child Neurology 23: 369–372

Smithells R W, Sheppard S, Schorah C J, Seller M J, Nevin N C, Harris R, Read A P, Fielding D W 1981 Apparent prevention of neural tube defects by periconceptional vitamin supplementation. Archives of Disease in Childhood 56: 911–918

*J.C.P. Weber*

# Limitations of a voluntary reporting system

It is seldom possible to predict adverse reactions to drugs on the basis of animal toxicology studies. If the animal studies demonstrate an unacceptable degree of toxicity, the drug does not reach the clinical trial stage, much less final marketing. It is therefore only possible to observe clinical situations when no serious animal toxicity has been demonstrated. There are numerous instances where severe adverse reactions have occurred under these circumstances leading to removal of the drug from the market. Conversely it is possible, with hindsight, to think of situations where there is teratogenesis in animals, but similar effects have not occurred in humans—corticosteroids are an example. Because of this inherent unreliability, toxicological studies can never take the place of careful clinical observation. Clinical trial results based on two to three thousand patients are often available when a product licence to market is sought. Experience of this extent will usually detect adverse reactions occurring with a frequency down to about 0.5 per cent. What it will not detect is a severe reaction, such as fatal liver necrosis, occurring at the rate of perhaps 1 in 20 000. It must be remembered that the expected number of such reactions in only 250 000 patients (a number very rapidly achieved after marketing of a commonly used drug) will be about 12.

A formal system of retrospective cohort monitoring known as 'Retrospective Assessment of Drug Safety' (RADS) would not produce an early warning of such a situation for reasons given later. It can only be detected by astute clinical observation and voluntary co-operation of doctors with both the Committee on Safety of Medicines and the appropriate pharmaceutical company. A recent instance of such a situation in the United States of America concerned the drug tienilic acid, an unusual diuretic with both antihypertensive and uricosuric properties. After marketing, voluntary reports from physicians to the Food and Drug Administration and to the manufacturers revealed an unacceptable incidence of hepatic damage. It was thus possible to stop further distribution of the drug within a few months of initial marketing and before huge numbers of patients had been exposed to it.

Systems which collect voluntary and anecdotal reports of suspected adverse reactions to drugs are less than perfect in operation. In the minds of some critics, there seems to be an idea that the voluntary reporting system could be replaced by some much more effective single system which would give an automatic and immediate warning of danger, or a complete reassurance of safety. Unfortunately, no such system exists, or is ever likely to exist.

It must be emphasised that monitoring the safety of drugs needs as many systems of surveillance, both immediate and applied, as may be necessary for the particular circumstances. The voluntary reporting system is seldom able to prove or disprove the culpability of a drug for a given adverse reaction, although the weight of evidence may sometimes permit an inference which is beyond reasonable doubt. One of the system's purposes is to allow a hypothesis, the confirmation or refutation of which may sometimes require carefully controlled prospective or retrospective studies. It is the purpose of this paper to show that, despite its limitations, a suitably supported voluntary reporting system is essential to a national drug monitoring centre.

**Disadvantages of the voluntary reporting system**

1. The association of the adverse reaction with the medicines prescribed must be recognisable to the reporter.
2. Not all adverse reactions are reported.
3. Reporting rates vary in relation to 'reminders' in current literature or in official publications.
4. The total population of patients at risk is unknown.
5. Reporting of a particular syndrome or symptom may be biased by some previous widely known incident with a related drug or with one used for similar treatment.

Medical recognition of the significance of a symptom or syndrome is an essential feature of any system, even including one in which 'clinical events' rather than adverse reactions are reported, and to which attention is drawn by their statistically significant predominance. Statistical examination will confirm the association, but medical interpretation must determine clinical significance.

The proportion of adverse reactions reported is, of course, impossible to determine with any certainty. Inman (1977) investigating the frequency of death due to aplastic anaemia in patients treated with phenylbutazone and oxyphenbutazone, found that only about 11 per cent had been reported to the Committee on Safety of Medicines.

Inman and Vessey (1968) found that in 1966 only 15 per cent of deaths due to thrombo-embolic complications in women taking oral contraceptives had been so reported. Because of such findings, the assumption is generally made that only about 10 per cent of adverse reactions are likely to be reported. This is a general order of magnitude, rather than a precise proportion, and the percentage varies considerably from one drug to another and at different times for the same drug. As an illustration, the yearly reporting rates of antibiotic associated colitis increased from 5 in 1973 to 44 in 1975 in response to reports in the literature, and to 71 in 1979 following an adverse reaction warning leaflet. On this occasion doctors were reminded that pseudomembranous colitis also occurred with antibiotics other than clindamycin and lincomycin. Reporting due to the other antibiotics rose subsequently from a yearly mean rate of 4 for the years 1973 to 1978, to 25 in 1979.

Lack of knowledge of the total population at risk prevents accurate calculations of incidence or prevalence. The number of patients exposed can sometimes be roughly calculated from consideration of prescribing figures derived from the Prescription Pricing Authority and their estimates of mean prescription size. Such calculations are crude at best, especially as they make no allowance for repeat prescriptions, and do not include hospital prescribing data. The figures can be more usefully used for comparative purposes between drugs of the same type used for the same clinical purpose.

Reporting may be completely biased by some previous adverse reactions experience. Thalidomide has produced such a situation with respect to relative over-reporting of limb reduction defects.

**Effective functions of the voluntary reporting system**

The following are the major functions of the system:

1. As an early warning generator.
2. To enable comparisons to be made with the adverse reaction pattern of similar drugs in other countries.
3. For in-depth studies.
4. To compare adverse reaction profiles of similar drugs used for the same clinical purpose.
5. To permit the setting up of hypotheses which may need testing by formal clinical studies.

As a producer of an early warning the system clearly depends on the ability of the reporting doctor to recognise the reaction and on his willingness to report it. Nevertheless, it is difficult to suggest any other system which could be relied on to perform this function notably more efficiently. Reporting of clinical events by RADS is delayed by the need to send out questionnaires after six months or one year of the clinical use of a drug, and by the subsequent delay of many months during which the questionnaires are returned, randomly sampled, computerised, analysed statistically and finally assessed medically. Such a system has little potential for early warning. The potential of the voluntary reporting system for an early warning can be increased by a greater awareness amongst doctors of the importance of reporting any unusual symptom in a patient taking a drug, especially a new drug, whether or not he thinks it to be a true adverse reaction. Attention should be particularly paid to affections of the organs of special sense, the haemopoietic system, the liver and kidneys and the central nervous system, and to any curious or unusual skin reaction. Had these principles been adhered to, it seems unlikely that the practolol syndrome would have escaped detection for four years. Interference with fetal and childhood dentition by tetracycline might possibly have been detected earlier than the 10 years it took in the absence of such a system.

Adverse reaction patterns can provide useful information to other national monitoring centres. United Kingdom experience of cimetidine proved useful to the Food and Drug Administration in the early days of the use of this drug in America, and useful exchanges of information often take place between the United Kingdom, Australia, and other World Health Organization member countries. Knowledge of the relative rates of prescribing of different drugs used for the same purpose can sometimes be of considerable value in obtaining a rough, but useful estimate of the relative frequency of a given adverse reaction. Total reports of pseudomembranous colitis for clindamycin, lincomycin and other antibiotics from 1973 to 1979, including peaks in reporting related to reminders, were: clindamycin 142; lincomycin 39; all other antibiotics 48. When this is corrected for the fact that clindamycin and lincomycin had a very small share of the total antibiotic market, it is not difficult to conclude that pseudomembranous colitis occurs more frequently with clindamycin than other antibiotics, despite the probability that there is still some degree of under-reporting with the latter.

Where a sufficient number of reports of a comparatively uncommon adverse reaction is available, as again in the case of antibiotic associated colitis, useful information on case-fatality rates in relation to age, the clinical condition for which the antibiotics were originally used, sex ratios of patients and other data can be obtained. Where it is desired to compare the pattern of adverse reactions between drugs of similar type used for the same clinical conditions, the adverse reaction profile, which is the number of reports of a particular type of adverse reaction expressed as a proportion of the total adverse reaction input for the drug concerned, is often useful. Similarly, to express a specific reaction as a proportion of a group of reactions may be revealing. If it had been possible to express limb reduction defects with thalidomide as a proportion of total skeletal abnormalities, and to compare this with that of other sedatives used in pregnancy, the specificity of thalidomide would have been sufficiently evident to demand investigation.

### Use of the voluntary reporting system in association with literature monitoring

Collectors of useful information do not always report it to the Committee on Safety of Medicines, sometimes preferring to publish their findings instead. This means that continuous monitoring of at least the major world medical journals must be an essential activity of a national drug monitoring centre. The Food and Drug Administration reviews about 140 publications every month. The computerised on-line facilities of Medline and other systems are available for this purpose and there are now some journals devoted entirely to abstracts of articles reporting adverse reactions.

The fact that a few adverse reactions have become the subject of a letter in a medical journal does not make them any more valid than the voluntary reporting system reports, but an entirely independent report in a situation where several similar unpublished reports already exist in the voluntary reporting system adds materially to the index of suspicion.

## VOLUNTARY REPORTING OF CONGENITAL ANOMALIES

It is in the field of congenital anomalies that the interpretation of voluntary reports must be handled most carefully. The antinauseant Debendox, containing doxylamine, dicyclomine and pyridoxine, recently received a great deal of sensational publicity because of some legal proceedings in the United States of America.

Debendox and other preparations containing antihistamines have been submitted to exhaustive investigations in epidemiological studies because of equivocal findings in animal teratology tests with certain antihistamines (surprisingly, not with doxylamine, despite some statements to the contrary). There have been numerous studies on Debendox. The Alberta study by Smith et al (1977) is particularly important since it was carried out as a retrospective case control study using 93 infants with limb reduction deformities and two separate carefully matched control groups. Suffice it to say that no scientifically acceptable evidence of an association between the consumption of Debendox or of other antinauseants containing antihistamines by pregnant women and congenital abnormalities in their offspring has emerged.

Examination of doctors' voluntary reports for Debendox for the period 1964 to December 1979, before the publicity, showed that there were 104 reports of congenital anomalies in the newborn of women who were taking Debendox at some stage of their pregnancies. Not all these reports were related to first trimester use, although many of them were because of the nature of the condition treated. In many, if not most, cases, other drugs had also been taken. No attempt has been made to confine the reports to those in which Debendox was the medicine particularly suspected by the notifying doctor. Reporting rates range from 1 to 16 per year, with a mean rate of 6.5 per year. The highest rate (of 16) was in 1977 and there was a small but statistically significant increase ($P < 0.05$) in the rates for 1977, 1978 and 1979.

It is pertinent at this stage to consider how many congenital abnormalities might have occurred in the total population of women exposed to Debendox, assuming that the rate was similar to that of all women. Of course it is not possible to know exactly how many women took Debendox in any particular year. Prescription Pricing Authority data suggest that the figure might be in excess of 350 000, but this is an overestimate because the figures give no information on repeated prescriptions. Reference to published papers shows an extraordinary variation in the proportion of pregnant women who took Debendox, from a level of a few per cent only to over 50 per cent in one American study. Communication with the manufacturers suggested that 20 per cent might not be too inaccurate in the United Kingdom. If we accept such a guess, then the population of women exposed to Debendox yearly must have been 20 per cent of the total number of births, so we are likely to be dealing with some figure of the general order of 120 000 in the United Kingdom. It is generally contended that congenital abnormalities of a severity likely to be recognisable at birth constitute at least 2 per cent of total births, so we would expect over 2000 of these to occur in our crudely calculated 'at risk' population. This annual figure must then be contrasted with the mean yearly rate of 6.5 reported by doctors under the voluntary system. It is clear that there must be a vast amount of underreporting and the few reports received presumably indicate a general belief that there is, in the overwhelming majority of cases, no relationship between the anomalies and the use of Debendox.

We have considered the total number of anomaly reports and it is necessary now to look at their quality or type. Here we encounter a surprising fact. Limb reduction deformities (which are held for the purpose of this paper to be either phocomelia or malformations involving absence of a limb or part of it or of digits) constitute no less than 42 per cent of the total number of reports. Is this an isolated phenomenon or does it apply to all other drugs? For example meclozine has 38 per cent of such reports and another antinauseant used in pregnancy, promethazine, has 12 per cent. Because of these curious findings it was thought necessary to consider for comparison both a medicine the use of which scarcely anyone would relate to a teratogenic hazard, and another which has come under some suspicion in this way. The drugs chosen were iron preparations (because they are used extensively in pregnancy) on the one hand, and norethisterone, and its combinations with ethinyloestradiol used as an oral contraceptive, on the other. In the case of iron the percentage of limb reduction defects was less than 5 and for the oral contraceptive 5.

It has not been possible to examine every drug in the adverse reactions register in this way but a superficial examination suggests that in doctors' reports, increases in limb reduction defects relate only to drugs used commonly to treat nausea and vomiting in pregnancy. In view of the epidemiological findings already referred to, it does not seem remotely likely that such a disproportion could be due to any true increase in incidence. The only other alternative is that it represents a reporting bias. We must now ask what percentage of specific abnormalities we would expect to find if they were drawn as fair samples from an unbiased population of congenital abnormalities of all kinds.

The Office of Population Censuses and Surveys in London collects information on congenital abnormalities from family doctors and midwives through District Health Authorities in England and Wales. This information, like that of the voluntary reporting system, is voluntarily supplied and is thought to represent about 40 per cent of the total (Weatherall J, personal communication). One of the reasons for the incompleteness of the data is that many minor abnormalities may go unrecognised at birth. Also, some major anomalies, especially those affecting the heart and great vessels, may not be diagnosed until later in life. Abnormalities easily recognisable at birth such as limb reduction defects, neural tube defects, hydrocephalus and cleft lip and palate are thought by the Office of Population Censuses and Surveys to be reported reasonably completely, and so published figures for the years 1975 to 1978 have been used to calculate percentages of these abnormalities, first in relation to total births for the year concerned. Limb reduction defects represent rather less than 2.5 per cent of total congenital abnormalities. This proportion, considering the crudity of the calculations, is not greatly different from the reported proportions for iron preparations and norethisterone (less than 5 per cent and 5 per cent respectively). It is markedly different from the high values reported for the anti-nauseants.

It would be valuable to determine whether the proportions of the two other groups of congenital abnormalities already mentioned are excessive also, or more closely related to expectation. The figures are given in Table 4.1. The rough expectations have been derived from the Office of Population Censuses and Surveys figures in the manner described for limb reduction defects. As will be seen from the Table, having regard to the very approximate nature of the calculations, there is no obvious difference in the general order of the proportions between the drugs or in relation to expectation. The proportions are very much what one would expect from random sampling.

**Table 4.1** Specific anomaly groups as percentages of total anomalies

| Congenital anomaly | Debendox | Norethisterone /ethinyloestradiol | Meclozine | Iron preparations | Expectation |
|---|---|---|---|---|---|
| Anencephaly, spina bifida, meningomyelocoele, hydrocephalus | 17 | 24 | 20 | 18 | 16 |
| Cleft lip or palate | 9 | | 6 | 10 | 7 |

None of the values differs greatly, bearing in mind the crudeness of the data, from the expected percentages derived from the population incidence, and there is no reason to suppose that any of these drugs is specifically related to the abnormalities cited.

Clearly then, disproportionately high reporting is confined to limb reduction defects. Finally, to put the matter into perspective, we should look at what sort of total numbers of specific abnormalities we might expect in our theoretical sample of 120 000 patients per year possibly exposed to treatment with Debendox. The figures for limb reduction defects, central nervous system defects as in the Table, and cleft lip or palate are respectively in excess of 50, 350 and 150. The mean number of these anomalies actually reported for the year 1975 to 1978 were, again respectively, 2, 1.5 and 1.3. Thus less than 4 per cent, 0.4 per cent and 0.9 per cent of what might have been possible totals for the three anomaly groups seem to have been reported. The actual value of these proportions is unimportant. What are important are the relative values. A situation in which a larger proportion of a particular anomaly is reported than of other more frequently occurring anomalies constitutes a reporting bias.

The hypothesis set up is therefore that the disproportion of reported limb reduction defects with antinauseants used to treat women in pregnancy is due to bias on the part of the reporting doctors. It should be noted that nothing is proved and that further evidence in the shape of the appropriate epidemiological studies already referred to is needed to confirm or refute such a hypothesis. The deductions on which it is based have been presented at some length to illustrate both the possible value and the limitations of the voluntary reporting system and the pitfalls which await the unwary user.

## FUNCTIONS OF THE COMMITTEE ON SAFETY OF MEDICINES

The Committee on Safety of Medicines has an unenviable task, and particularly so in an era of increasingly vociferous criticism from sections of the public, from Parliament and from what is loosely generally known as 'the media'. If the Committee acts quickly, banning or limiting the use of a drug on the strength of a few serious or fatal adverse reactions it is criticised by the medical profession, a few of whom may have obtained good results with the drug and have been lucky enough to have avoided the reactions concerned. If it waits to gain further experience because the balance of evidence is insufficient for immediate action other than perhaps a mention in its bulletin *Current Problems*, and more cases occur, it is criticised by the media for not acting quickly enough. It may be subjected to pressure by groups seeking financial recompense, by those who benefit in various ways from associated litigation and by others who seek to score political points from the discomfiture of a ministerially approved committee. If it seeks to ban a drug of long standing which has produced a formidable series of relatively severe though non-fatal adverse reactions, in a situation where other quite adequate treatment is available, then it may find itself arraigned by both the profession and the pharmaceutical industry; the one on the grounds that their choice of treatment is threatened and the other that the drug is unique and that all other similar drugs produce the same adverse reactions which have, for some reason, not been reported.

Data considered by the Committee is collated and researched carefully by senior doctors usually specialised either in clinical medicine, clinical pharmacology or related medical sciences and often also with experience of pharmaceutical industrial practice. These data, and the recommendations of the medical assessors, are debated by an appropriate sub-committee containing members versed in toxicology, pharmacology, epidemiology and medical statistics and representing several medical specialties. Recommendations of the sub-committee are subsequently considered by the main Committee which suggests a course of action to the Licensing Authority. There are routes of appeal open to pharmaceutical companies wishing to dispute the Committee's recommendations, with the ultimate possibility of referral (in the case of a medical or pharmaceutical issue) to the Medicines Commission. Action of a regulatory kind is therefore taken only after most careful deliberation. The system, like any other, is not devoid of faults, but it appears to compare favourably with those used by other socially advanced countries and should remain an essential adjunct to other methods described.

## REFERENCES

Inman W H W 1977 Study of fetal bone marrow depression with special reference to phenylbutazone and oxyphenbutazone. British Medical Journal i: 1500–1505

Inman W H W, Vessey M P 1968 Investigation of deaths from pulmonary, coronary, and cerebral thrombosis and embolism in women of child-bearing age. British Medical Journal ii: 193–199

Smith E S O, Dafoe C S, Miller J R, Banister P 1977 An epidemiological study of congenital reduction deformities of the limbs. British Journal of Preventive and Social Medicine 31: 39–41

# 5 Prescribing in pregnancy

*D.F. Hawkins*

We have considered the fact that nearly all drugs must be viewed as capable of passing the placenta and reaching the fetus. The few that do not pass, heparin for example, are still potentially capable of affecting the fetus by their action on the mother and the placenta. The fact that testing of drugs in animals has limited applicability to human pregnancy and may produce misleading results has been brought out. The great majority of perinatal toxicological studies seem to be intended to convey medicolegal protection to the pharmaceutical houses and political protection to the official regulatory bodies, rather that to produce information that might be of value in human therapeutics. Some of the major difficulties encountered in demonstrating teratogenic effects in humans have been reviewed. When the complexity of the concept of causation of a fetal abnormality in this context is added to the very considerable methodological problems of demonstrating low level associations between the use of drugs and hazards to the fetus, interpretation in definitive scientific terms becomes extremely difficult except with a very few agents. When it comes to early recognition of hazards in pregnancy of drugs newly introduced into human therapeutics, sampling problems are added to the difficulty of demonstrating a causal association by epidemiological methods. Although there are techniques for overcoming some of these problems, the results must be at most suggestive.

These difficulties are scientific in nature, being concerned with the derivation and dissemination of basic factual information. The problems of prescribing in pregnancy are compounded by other considerations.

**The ethical problem** (see Hawkins 1982).
The intention of management in pregnancy is to achieve a healthy mother and a healthy baby. During pregnancy, the mother's health is the primary consideration, because if it is not maintained the baby is at risk. Prescriptions in pregnancy are therefore intended to

contribute to maternal health with the minimum risk to the baby from the side effects of treatment. If treating a maternal condition conveys a specifiable risk to the baby, then two processess should take place before it is initiated. The doctor should first specify the risk and give an opinion as to its magnitude, together with his advice as to whether or not the treatment proposed is orthodox, reasonable and in the patient's best interests. Secondly, the patient must make a value judgement as to whether or not she accepts the advice.

The extent to which these matters should be pursued, and the emphasis which should be given to the discussion are related both to the actual magnitude of the risk and to any publicity which may have been given to it by the news media. Some agents such as oral iron or vitamins have been given after 10 weeks of pregnancy to many millions of women over several decades without any hazard being specified; it should suffice to state that the tablets are harmless to the fetus. Other drugs, such as anti-emetics, may be equally harmless, but have been subjected to attacks in the news media or in the courts. It then becomes necessary to go into considerable detail with the patient, not only to indicate the extent of the evidence and the weight of opinion that the drug is harmless, but also to suggest the potential hazards of not using it. It may well be indicated that the consequences of uncontrolled vomiting may be more harmful than any undetectably small risk that might be associated with use of anti-emetic drugs.

When there are some grounds to suspect a small risk, a different orientation is appropriate. It is reasonable to indicate that any woman undertaking a pregnancy is susceptible to a risk of 1 in 50 of having a grossly abnormal baby, but it is unreasonable to put it in these words, which represent the epidemiological viewpoint of a doctor. From the patient's perspective the prognosis is 50 to 1 that her baby is going to be essentially normal. With corticosteroid treatment in pregnancy, if there is any risk of cleft palate in humans—and that is by no means clear—the added risk is represented by odds of at least 100 to 1 that the baby will be unaffected by the drugs in this respect (Sidhu and Hawkins 1981). With medical conditions requiring corticosteroids in pregnancy the chances that the fetus would be deleteriously affected by withdrawing the drugs are considerable. Similarly, with an epileptic patient under treatment during pregnancy there is a 6 per cent risk of a major fetal abnormality (Smithells 1976). From the patient's viewpoint the odds are 17 to 1 that her baby will be normal and these can probably be considerably improved by folic acid supplements and anticonvulsant dose adjustment initiated before pregnancy. In some contrast to the healthy patient, who may be alarmed at the mere mention of the subject of congenital abnormality, there is seldom difficulty in conveying hard statistical facts of this sort to women with major medical disorders. They have usually taken the potential risks of pregnancy into account before conceiving and have already made their value judgements. What they want to hear is how the dangers can be reduced to a minimum, and it is to this that the doctor's attention will be directed.

When the problem is one of malignant disease in pregnancy then it is first essential that the doctor has his facts right. For example carcinoma of the breast can be treated by mastectomy and radiotherapy in pregnancy without serious hazard to the baby, and the notion that recurrence of the disease is more likely in pregnancy than in other women of the same age group was dispelled many years ago. Cytotoxic drugs used for treating leukaemia of course have a risk of causing fetal abnormality, but with some of the drugs, particularly busulphan and mercaptopurine, the risk may not be unacceptable even if they are continued through the first trimester. Sometimes treatment can be altered to cope with the problem of early pregnancy; leucophoresis may be used. In the second and third trimesters the cytotoxic drugs seem to be relatively harmless to the fetus (Sweet and Kinzie 1976). It is essential that the best estimate of the hazard involved be presented to the patients. If they are unacceptable to her, then she has the ethical right to abortion.

**Medicolegal considerations**

It is possible for a doctor to be sued in civil law for negligently prescribing a medicine which led to abortion or intra-uterine death of the fetus. The reason why such an action is unlikely is that very few drugs are known which could reasonably be taken to have caused an abortion. If such agents were available, they would be used for procuring legal abortion. For example, supposing a doctor were to prescribe an ergot preparation for migraine in pregnancy and the patient subsequently aborted. Innumerable cases would be produced where such treatment had been given to pregnant women without harm, and irrefutable evidence would be produced that a proportion of pregnant women undergo abortion spontaneously. The two groups of drugs which can cause abortion, prostaglandins and cytotoxic drugs, are most unlikely to be prescribed negligently.

On the other hand, the Congenital Disabilities (Civil Liability) Act 1976 does give a reason for concern. Under this Act, if a child is born disabled as a result of wrongful prescription of a drug during the pregnancy, then the doctor who prescribed the drug is liable.

The key clause to this Act is that the doctor is 'not answerable to the child for anything he did . . . if he took reasonable care having due regard to then received professional opinion applicable to the particular class of case'. It is clear that the Act was intended to protect doctors who prescribe in good faith, in what they reasonably believe to be the best interests of their patients. The actions of pharmaceutical houses is making such statements as 'should not be given during pregnancy' about many drugs where there is not a shred of evidence that they are harmful to the fetus (Data Sheet Compendium 1981-1982), are irresponsible in this context. The statements are made, with the tacit approval of the Committee on Safety of Medicines, in the hope that they might confer legal protection on the companies concerned if changes in product liability law leave them open to accusations of contributing to a congenital abnormality. The fact that the statements could be quoted to the detriment of doctors who are using the drugs in the best interests of their patients seems to be of no concern.

Similar considerations apply to such authoritarian pronouncements such as made by the Committee on the Review of Medicines (1979) about barbiturates. The Committee included pregnancy as a contraindication to the use of these drugs, without reasoning, evidence or documentation. The opinion was given that benzodiazepines are safer, efficacious alternative preparations. It is said the word 'contraindication' does not mean that the drug must not be used in pregnancy. This is technically true—the Shorter Oxford English Dictionary says 'an indication which "makes against" a particular treatment'—but general interpretation will be in terms of the common use of the word. It is also said that the pronouncement carried no medicolegal weight. This is patently untrue—in the United Kingdom it could well be taken as an expression of 'received professional opinion' under the Congenital Disabilities Act. The weight of opinion of many obstetricians who have needed to use barbiturates as sedatives and anticonvulsants in pregnancy for many years and have not seen harm resulting, is considerable. This is particularly important as, only two years later, neonatal paediatricians are expressing concern at the time for which maternally administered benzodiazepines are retained in newborn babies, and are asking obstetricians to use barbiturates instead!

**Vested interests**

Note may be taken of the fact that Debendox was the most widely used anti-emetic, having been given to over thirty million pregnant women over 23 years, when the news media, medicolegal and even

Parlimentary, campaigns to suggest it was teratogenic were undertaken. Similarly, the coincidence between the representations made to the Food and Drug Administration in the United States of America that metronidazole might be teratogenic and the introduction of this enormously successful oral trichomonacide to the American market will be noted. The sceptic will also consider that manufacture of barbiturates is today an unprofitable commercial proposition, whilst many hundreds of millions of pounds have been made from marketing benzodiazepines. Whilst the individuals and organisations who have added most fuel to the flames intended to consume the use of these drugs are above suspicion, the questing mind is led to ponder on the subtlety of commercial influences on the practice of medicine. Such thoughts are of course only undertaken in the same spirit of scientific curiosity which led to the unjustified speculations on teratogenic potential.

**Patient motivation**

Ingestion of drugs is often cited and exploited by patients requesting legal abortion. If the request is persistent after the negligible or very small magnitude of risk has been explained, there is usually another reason why the patient wants the pregnancy terminated. This may sometimes be obvious to the doctor without being perceived by the patient. Abortions are often performed on the grounds of potential teratogenesis, when the real grounds are the patient's anxiety. It is unwise to condone such a course of action. In a recent case (Medical Defence Union 1979), a subfertile woman had a hysterosalpingogram performed at a time when she was subsequently determined to have had an early pregnancy. The pregnancy was terminated 'because of the irradiation risk to the fetus'. In fact there has been no valid demonstration in humans of any risk associated with such a dose of radiation. According to Sternberg (1973), 50 rad (0.5 Gy) is the minimum dose at which there can be considered to be a clear association with fetal damage. The invalidity of the grounds for terminating the pregnancy passed unnoticed. They were taken as the basis for awarding damages to the patient on the grounds that failure to exclude the pregnancy led to an unnecessary termination of pregnancy. It must be made abundantly clear in cases like this, when the real risk to the fetus from a physical agent or ingested drugs is insubstantial, that the reason for performing a legal abortion is the patient's anxiety.

It was estimated by Wilson in 1973 that only 10 per cent of congenital abnormalities have an identified environmental cause which in some cases is a drug. Even so ,the woman who has had an abnormal baby often has an emotional need to find something other than her own episode of reproductive insufficiency to blame for the outcome of her pregnancy. In addition, she may have the practical need for financial support for a disabled child. Though sympathy for these needs may seem appropriate, it is quite unreasonable for responsible doctors to lend support to contentions of an association with drug use of which there has been no valid demonstration.

## PRINCIPLES OF PRESCRIBING IN PREGNANCY

Faced with such factual inadequacies, compounded by emotional overlay and medicolegal implications, one could almost generate sympathy for the practitioner who refused to prescribe any drugs for pregnant women. On the other hand such an attitude would undoubtedly endanger the health and even the lives of some of his patients. Harm to the fetus resulting from omission of treatment is specifically mentioned in the Congenital Disabilities Act as giving rise to liability.

Fortunately, adherence to the basic rules of prescribing, sensible policies with respect to drug use and reasonable interpretation of any risks to patients, protect the very great majority of practitioners from either causing harm to a fetus or being accused of so doing.

The basic rules are simple: (see Hawkins 1982)

1. Review all patients with medical disorders before they conceive, regarding every women of reproductive age as a potential antenatal patient, and encouraging them to attend for preconceptional counselling before embarking on planned pregnancies.
2. Question the real need for any drug whose prescription in pregnancy is proposed, and give due consideration to alternative modes of treatment.
3. Review all drug regimens in pregnancy to see how careful therapeutics and good control can minimise risks.
4. Use agents which have been widely employed in pregnancy for years in preference to the latest drugs.

### Prescribing policies

Confusion can be caused by failure to distinguish appropriate prescribing policies from hazards to individual patients. For example, it has become an accepted policy in recent years to withhold prophylactic oral iron from patients during the first 12 or 14 weeks of pregnancy. This probably arose partly from Nelson and Forfar's (1971) survey, which suggested that there might be an association between iron given in the first few weeks and congenital malformations. This result was probably due to retrospective bias and many subsequent studies have failed to confirm any association; see, for example the prospective study of the Royal College of General Practitioners (1975). Obstetricians have seldom bothered to comment on the policy for two reasons. Firstly, it is doubtful if iron supplements are necessary or even desirable in pregnancy if the patient is not anaemic. Secondly, iron tablets are a major cause of nausea and vomiting in pregnancy and can easily exacerbate morning sickness if given in the first trimester. It will be clear that it is quite wrong to consider there is any teratogenic risk to a patient who has taken iron in the first trimester.

Another example occurs with women who become pregnant whilst taking an oral contraceptive—by no means as rare an occurrence as the advertisers would have us believe. There probably is a slightly increased risk of congenital abnormality, particularly if the fetus is male (see Darling and Hawkins 1981, for review). It is therefore an important policy to exclude pregnancy before a patient with infrequent menstruation or amenorrhoea starts taking a contraceptive pill, and to discontinue the oral contraceptive promptly if a patient taking it unexpectedly misses a menstrual period. On the other hand, from the perspective of a patient who conceives whilst using oral contraception, the risk of a drug-associated fetal abnormality is very small indeed, probably between 1 in 500 and 1 in 5000. This can not be considered a serious risk justifying legal abortion.

Metronidazole has been accused of being teratogenic, though the experimental work on which these accusations were based has been shown to be defective, and there is ample evidence that the drug is not teratogenic in humans (see Morgan 1978). To postpone treatment of asymptomatic vaginal trichomoniasis until the second trimester is nonetheless a reasonable policy, on the general principle of avoiding unnecessary drugs in early pregnancy. To neglect treatment, because she is pregnant, of a patient in whom trichomoniasis is causing symptoms is indefensible, when the absence of harm to the fetus has been demonstrated in many thousands of women.

## Classification of drugs with respect to teratogenesis

When drug treatment is to be used in pregnancy, a simple classification (Hawkins 1981) provides guidelines.

*Major teratogens in humans* may be defined as agents whose use in pregnancy conveys a proved and considerable risk of causing a congenital abnormality. Apart from thalidomide, examples are few, but some cytotoxic drugs and radiochemicals fall in this class, so do the tetracyclines, even though their known effect is only on primary dentition. Only very exceptional circumstances should indicate prescription of these drugs in pregnancy. With the exception of tetracyclines, the pregnant woman who has been exposed to them during a susceptible phase of pregnancy has a clear case for legal abortion.

*Therapeutic agents with a known risk* include a range of drugs necessary to the health of women with medical disorders. The hazard is usually small, with an excellent chance of a healthy baby, but the problem must be discussed with the patient. With nearly all these agents choice of alternative drugs, careful control of dose and use of supplementary agents such as folic acid can minimise the risk.

*Agents which have been accused* of having a teratogenic risk on anecdotal or insubstantial experimental or theoretical grounds are legion. Many of them have been exonerated with the aid of extensive clinical trials. Nonetheless, when an alternative drug of similar efficacy, which has been used for a long time without being so accused , is available, the careful practitioner will be inclined to use it.

*Drugs which have been adequately demonstrated to be completely harmless to the fetus* are the exception. Even though the demonstration has been one which must be accepted as beyond reasonable doubt, the possibility that an association with some imponderable factor could cause harm to the baby of one woman in many thousands can never be completely excluded. Adherence to the rule of not prescribing a drug without an adequate indication will provide ample protection for the practitioner.

## REFERENCES

Committee on the Review of Medicines 1979 Recommendations on barbiturate preparations. British Medical Journal ii: 719–720

Congenital Disabilities (Civil Liability) Act 1976 Her Majesty's Stationary Office, London

Darling M R, Hawkins D F 1981 Sex hormones in pregnancy. In: Wood S M, Beeley L (editors): Prescribing in pregnancy. Clinics in Obstetrics and Gynaecology 8 (2): 405–419.

Data Sheet Compendium 1981–82. Datapharm Publications, London

Hawkins D F 1981 Effects of drugs in pregnancy and during lactation. In: Roberts D F, Chester R (editors) Changing patterns of conception and fertility. Academic Press, London, pp. 135–163

Hawkins D F 1983 Ethical and medical considerations in the use of drugs in pregnancy. In: Kuemmerle H P (editor) Drug therapy in pregnancy. Georg Thieme, Stuttgart, (in press)

Medical Defence Union 1979 Annual Report. London, p.24

Morgan I F D 1978 Metronidazole treatment in pregnancy. International Journal of Gynaecology and Obstetrics 15: 501–507

Nelson M M, Forfar J O 1971 Associations between drugs administered during

pregnancy and congenital abnormalities of the fetus. British Medical Journal: 523–527
Royal College of General Practitioners 1975 Morbidity and drugs in pregnancy. Journal of the Royal College of General Practitioners 25: 631–645
Sidhu R K, Hawkins D F 1981 Corticosteroids. In: Wood S M, Beeley L (editors) Prescribing in pregnancy. Clinics in Obstetrics and Gynaecology 8 (2): 383–404
Smithells R W 1976 Environmental teratogens of man. British Medical Bulletin 32: 27–33
Sternberg J 1973 Radiation risk in pregnancy. Clinical Obstetrics and Gynecology 16 (1): 235 –278
Sweet D L, Kinzie J 1976 Consequences of radiotherapy and antineoplastic therapy for the fetus. Journal of Reproductive Medicine 17: 241–246
Wilson J G 1973 Present status of drugs as teratogens in man. Teratology 7: 3–15

# Section two

# 6 The therapeutics of normal pregnancy

*D. F. Hawkins*

The majority of abnormal conceptions undergo spontaneous abortion in the first few weeks of pregnancy. Of pregnancies that survive the first trimester, between 1 and 3 per cent result in a baby with a major congenital malformation. An additional 3 to 6 per cent of babies have minor abnormalities recognisable at birth, the exact figures depending on the definition of abnormality. How many have functional characteristics which may be thought to deviate sufficiently from the average to be regarded as 'abnormal' is not known. Wilson (1973) estimated that only some 2 to 3 per cent of human malformations are drug associated. The basis of his calculations is open to question, but even assuming a twofold underestimate , only 1 in 1000 pregnancies would result in a drug associated major congenital abnormality.

If the problem of environmental factors which contribute to abnormality in children is to be reduced, iatrogenic factors should be amongst the first to be considered, even though they may have a relatively small role. All the procedures employed in antenatal management merit consideration, not just the prescription of drugs.

## ANTENATAL PREPARATION

Preconceptional counselling has little to contribute, from a medical point of view, for the average healthy woman in a developed country. The only function that can be served is educational, providing information on the anatomy and physiology of pregnancy and answering queries; perhaps relieving anxieties, perhaps creating them. On the other hand, for women with a problem such as obesity, smoking or maternal age, for those who have had previous spontaneous abortions or perinatal losses, and for those with medical complications, including hypertension, heart disease and diabetes, preconceptional counselling is very important with respect to the success of the next pregnancy. Similarly, in undeveloped countries and communities where nutrition is inadequate and general health problems are common, it is highly desirable to review women intending to conceive in advance, and try to improve their general health and nutrition before they embark on the first trimester of pregnancy. In these contexts preconceptional counselling can now contribute to the prevention of congenital abnormality and pregnancy losses.

Recently, a lot of attention has been paid to early antenatal attendance as soon as pregnancy is suspected. In practice there is little the obstetrician can do for the healthy woman at this stage and most specialist practitioners find it more helpful to see the average patient at 12 weeks. There may be an advantage to seeing the woman with complications before this, but the potential for a constructive contribution is not so great as it is at a preconceptional visit.

Antenatal classes can be of educational value, and undoubtedly can contribute to the general welfare and happiness of pregnant women. Objective benefits are more difficult to establish and there is no good evidence that 'relaxation exercises', 'psychoprophylaxis' or any of the other techniques modify the actual process of labour or requirement for analgesia. A few women may become depressed if the benefits claimed fail to materialise, developing a sense of failure. Overindulgence in the pelvic rocking exercises described by Heardman (1959) can lead to strain of the maternal lumbosacral and sacro-iliac joints. The hyperventilation of 'breathing exercises' can lead to tetany, but Moya et al (1965) observed little relationship between whether or not the mother was urged to hyperventilate and the actual development of maternal alkalosis. The only two cases they found with alkalosis sufficient to harm the babies, who became acidotic, were both being artificially ventilated under general anaesthesia. Theoretically, breath-holding during uterine contractions in labour can lead to fetal hypoxia but there is no evidence that this actually occurs.

Hypnotic techniques convey two risks. If the suggestion is implanted that pain will cease, it must be accompanied by the suggestion that uterine contractions will continue, or uterine inertia will result. The obstetrician must be scrupulous in looking for obstructed labour. Under hypnotic suggestion uterine rupture can occur without the usual symptoms and signs.

The Leboyer (1975) approach consists of delivery in a quiet dark room, avoidance of stimulation of the baby, placing it on the mother's abdomen, delaying clamping of the cord, and then gently massaging the baby and giving it a warm bath. The randomised clinical trial conducted by Nelson et al (1980) detected no objective advantages to the baby, and only to the mother in that her perception of the baby's behaviour when it was 8 months old was improved. The regimen is harmless provided it is modified in three respects. It is essential that the obstetrician has enough light to see clearly what he is doing and to make an adequate appraisal of the condition of the baby. Failure to extract mucus from the baby's mouth, nose and pharynx, or to prevent hypothermia when it is placed on the mother's abdomen, can predispose to neonatal chest infections, perhaps related to inhalation of debris (Kavvos J, personal communication 1980). Only when the obstetrician is satisfied as to the condition of the baby and it is dry and warm should it be given to the mother.

Husbands in the labour ward are no more a source of infection than hospital personnel. The last major outbreak of group A streptococcal infections in a maternity unit in the United States of America was traced to a spot on an anaesthetist's hand (Jewett et al 1968), and the common site for group B streptococcal carriage is the vagina.

## DIET IN PREGNANCY

Attention to the potential role of dietary factors in relation to fetal welfare is increasing. The recent concern in America about the possible ill-effects of caffeine (Morris and Weinstein 1981) is typical. There is no evidence that intake of coffee or tea is teratogenic in humans. In interpreting data in this context, obstetricians should beware of arbitrary lists of nutritional requirements in pregnancy, such as those given by the Department of Health and Social Security (1979) in Great Britain. For example, we recently surveyed 41 unselected patients not receiving dietary supplements at their first visit to the antenatal clinic. Daily intake of folate varied from 106 to 602 μg. Only two patients were ingesting the Department of Health's recommended allowance of 500 μg/day; but only one of the 41 patients had a subnormal serum folate level of just below 3 μg/l. Forty-eight unselected, unsupplemented patients had vitamin D intakes of between 0.2 and 7.9 μg of cholecalciferol, all well below the recommended 10 μg (400 i.u.) daily. Only one of these had a serum 25-hydroxy vitamin D level below 4 μg/l, warranting further investigation; she was from the Middle East.

In a developed country, the only dietary advice needed by healthy women with no relevant abnormal obstetric history and no dietary fads is to control their calorie intake if they start gaining weight excessively.

## Calorie intake

Statistically speaking, the best prognosis for pregnancy occurs when the patient is the correct weight for her height at the start of pregnancy and gains between 7 and 9 kg during the pregnancy (Nyirjesy et al 1968). The fact that heavier women who gain more tend to produce larger babies (Niswander et al 1969) does not imply a better obstetric outcome.

Calorie intake can only be assessed in terms of weight gain during the pregnancy. Individual variation is so great that an arbitrary level is meaningless. The best time for assessment is the middle trimester, when morning sickness is over and reduced weight gain or actual loss which may result from placental insufficiency has not started. It is by no means clear that fetal welfare can be improved by altering the calorie intake of women with an abnormal weight gain. The evidence (Hamlin 1952, 1953) that weight control can reduce the incidence of toxaemia has been widely questioned. On the other hand good nutrition with a weight gain of 7 to 9 kg in pregnancy is compatible with maternal health and a low perinatal mortality.

Gross obesity is associated with a high perinatal mortality. In patients weighing more than 100 kg at the start of pregnancy, the outlook for the fetus can be improved by actual weight reduction during pregnancy.

Weight control in pregnancy is best achieved through dietary advice alone, though there is some evidence that the appetite suppressant fenfluramine is not teratogenic. Data on similar drugs in human pregnancy is sparse.

## Protein, fat and carbohydrate

In developed countries it is unusual to find intakes of less than 60 g of protein daily in pregnant women. Adolescent girls who require protein for their own growth, women of Asian extraction who sometimes have a low protein intake, and vegetarians, may benefit from advice. All three groups have an increased incidence of dysmature babies, and may produce somewhat larger babies if they eat more protein. The actual amounts of fat and carbohydrate in the diet seem to have little relevance to fetal welfare except insofar as they relate to total calorie consumption.

## Fluids

Fluid intake *per se* should not be restricted in the pregnant woman. Hypotonus and stasis in the lower urinary tract predisposes to infection if fluid excretion is reduced. Most of the oedema seen in pregnancy is either physiological and harmless or associated with pre-eclampsia, the management then being that of toxaemia. In some patients with heart failure and those with carpal tunnel syndrome, the correct management is with carefully controlled use of thiazide diuretics, not restriction of fluid intake.

The aspect of fluid intake which may require attention is related to the nature of the fluids. A patient may gain weight excessively because of intake of sweetened or alcoholic drinks, and need advice to take low calorie drinks instead. Certainly, intake of alcoholic fluids should not exceed the equivalent of 90 ml ethanol a day, or there is a serious risk of the fetal alcohol syndrome, and more than 30 ml ethanol a day may be associated with intra-uterine growth retardation.

## Minerals

An average diet contains between 5 and 10 g of sodium chloride a day. The concept of salt restriction during pregnancy has been abandoned, except for selected patients with essential hypertension where the blood pressure is salt sensitive. It is now accepted that the original results of de Snoo (1937), who thought that the incidence of pre-eclampsia was reduced by salt restriction, were due to other factors in antenatal care. Robinson (1958) showed that high salt diets do not cause pre-eclampsia and in fact some patients with this complication improve. Bower (1964) gave patients salt intakes of 1.5 to 25 g/day without any effect on toxaemia.

Basic daily dietary requirements of pregnant women are said to include calcium (1.2 g), magnesium (0.45 g), phosphorus (1.2 g) and iodine (125 μg). Milk alone contains 0.12 g of calcium, 0.01 g of magnesium and 0.1 g of phosphorus per 100 g and an ordinary mixed diet is unlikely to be deficient. There is a small chance that diets rich in oatmeal, which contains the calcium binder phytic acid, may restrict calcium absorption. Otherwise, calcium and magnesium are only likely to be deficient in malabsorption syndromes or after parathyroidectomy. Calcium lactate tablets, taken in the pious hope that they may relieve nocturnal leg cramps in pregnancy, seem to be harmless. On the other hand, excessive intake of iodine, in proprietary cough medicines, has been reported to give rise to neonatal goitre and hypothyroidism (Carswell et al 1970).

*Iron.* Total body iron in a healthy woman is about 3.5 g. The physiological cost of iron in a pregnancy has been estimated, allowing for the amenorrhoea, as some 550 mg required for the formation of the fetus and placenta. Scott (1979) would double this, including 500 mg attributed to increased maternal red cell mass, though this will eventually go back into the iron stores. Adding the average total daily iron loss of about 1.5 mg, the pregnant woman needs to absorb some 5 mg of iron daily to maintain her iron stores. The daily intake of dietary iron in our West London population of very mixed origins varies from 6 to 26 mg/day.

It follows that most women are capable of maintaining their iron stores through pregnancy by eating a normal unsupplemented diet. Even if absorption is somewhat impaired, they can cope without developing anaemia, at the expense of the iron stores. From this point of view it is only women who are anaemic or have depleted iron stores at the start of pregnancy, perhaps due to chronic nutritional deficiency, menorrhagia or repeated pregnancies, who need routine iron supplements. Those who are anaemic are easily identified with a haemoglobin estimation performed at a preconceptional or antenatal clinic, and require investigation and appropriate treatment, generally with iron and folic acid. To detect those with deficient iron stores with reasonable accuracy requires estimation of plasma ferritin (Kelly et al 1977).

What then, is the case for giving routine iron supplements in pregnancy? Thirty years ago in Glasgow, 20 per cent of women had haemoglobins below 10 g/dl at some time in pregnancy (Scott and Govan 1949). Today, in developed countries, even in poor urban communities, due to improved health, nutrition and social and economic circumstances, as well as spacing of pregnancies, anaemia is much less common. In West London, haemoglobins of 10 g/dl are only found in 1 to 2 per cent of women at their first antenatal attendance, although the dietary iron intakes of two-thirds of them are below the Department of Health and Social Security's (1979) recommendation of 13 mg/day.

Iron supplementation is said to prevent the fall in haemoglobin of 0.5 to 1.0 g/dl which often occurs physiologically during pregnancy, due to retention of fluid in the intravascular compartment, increased blood volume and haemodilution. It is far from clear if iron supplements have this effect. In our own studies the haemoglobins of women with anaemia at the start of pregnancy rose in response to oral iron; those with high haemoglobins at the start still demonstrated the physiological anaemia. It only needs a few very mildly anaemic women in these groups treated to respond to iron and the *average* fall in haemoglobin is reduced, even though the healthiest women still develop the physiological anaemia. It is doubtful if any purpose is served by apparently combating the physiological anaemia in these women (Lind et al 1975). With the doses of oral iron formerly used a few cases of macrocytic anaemia were generated (Taylor and Lind, 1976), probably due to stimulation of haemopoeisis in situations where folic acid absorption was impaired. If iron is used prophylactically in pregnancy, it should be accompanied by small doses of folic acid (350 μg/day). It is said that iron is cheap. If a simple preparation of iron and folic acid was used for 6 months of every pregnancy in Great Britain the cost would be about £1 million. With the more complex proprietary preparations commonly prescribed by family practitioners, this may rise to as much as £5 million. (Hawkins 1981). Finally, it is said that women given prophylactic iron in pregnancy and their babies are healthier. There is no objective evidence for this (Hemminki and Starfield 1978). In spite of clinical trials purporting to show the contrary, there is no doubt that iron preparations often cause gastro-intestinal disturbances. They have been said to be the commonest cause of vomiting in pregnancy, and their tendency to give rise to constipation or diarrhoea frequently results in the patient ceasing to take them.

Although Nelson and Forfar's (1971) retrospective study suggested a possible association between oral iron given in the first few weeks of pregnancy and a low incidence of fetal abnormality, this was not confirmed in the Royal College of General Practitioners' prospective study (1975). Nonetheless, obstetricians do not object to the avoidance of oral iron administration during the first trimester, while morning sickness may be a problem.

Prophylactic oral iron is probably unnecessary for the majority of healthy pregnant women in a developed country. If there is felt to be an indication for prophylaxis, iron and folic acid tablets containing 100 mg of elemental iron as fumarate and 0.35 mg of folic acid, one daily taken with the main meal, is as good as more expensive proprietary preparations. Iron deficiency anaemia in pregnancy is often associated with defective absorption and should be treated with iron and folic acid, 5 mg daily, to overcome the absorption defect.

*Lead.* It has been considered that chronic lead poisoning contributed materially to the decline and fall of the Roman Empire by causing impotence, sterility, abortion, stillbirth and premature labour, as well as mental retardation in children (Gilfillan 1965). Lead-lined vessels are no longer used for storing wine or preserved fruit and cases of plumbism from contaminated water are very rare. Nonetheless, concern has been expressed about the possible ill-effects of dietary lead from tinned food and shellfish, and the fact that the level of lead in tap water in some British cities has been reported to exceed the World Health Organization recommended limits (Bryce-Smith and Waldron 1974). It has been suggested that levels of lead in the bones of stillborn babies are increased (Bryce-Smith et al 1977).

The maximum safe level for lead in water is said to be 0.25 μmol/l (50 μg/l). In pregnant women a blood lead level should be below 1.5 μmol/l (300 μg/l). Levels of 2.0 μmol/l (400 μg/l) or more are indicative of excessive intake. In West London blood lead levels in healthy antenatal patients range from 0.4 to 0.7 μmol/l (90 to 140 μg/l). Bryce-Smith and Stephens (1981) have suggested that levels of greater than 0.25 μmol/l (50μg/l) might be considered abnormal and that the great majority of pregnant women and children are under the adverse influences of lead. This view must be regarded as extreme.

*Other trace elements* are of little general importance in the present context. The subject has been reviewed by Moghissi (1981).

## Vitamins

Clinical trials of vitamin supplementation in pregnancy were reviewed by Hemminki and Starfield (1978). They could find little objective evidence of any benefit to mother or baby, with the possible exception of the use of pyridoxine supplements. This vitamin, given in the form of lozenges (7 mg, 3 times a day) appeared to reduce the development of maternal dental caries in pregnancy (Hillman et al 1962). Its use might be considered reasonable in environments where the incidence of dental problems in pregnancy is troublesome.

Dietary surveys of pregnant women often show apparent deficiencies of intake of particular vitamins, compared to Department of Health and Social Security (1979) recommendations. It must be recognised that recommended levels are largely arbitrary, and in the absence of evidence that they do any good routine administration to healthy women in developed countries cannot be advised.

## Special groups of antenatal patients

*Folic acid.* It has been known for a long time that certain patients are at particular risk for developing megaloblastic anaemia in pregnancy and that this could be prevented by giving them folic acid supplements. They include women with depleted iron stores such as those with menorrhagia and grande multiparae, who need extra folic acid to cope with the haemopoeitic response to the oral iron they will be given; women with deficient absorption, perhaps suggested by anaemia in a previous pregnancy; those taking drugs such as anti-convulsants, antimalarials, co-trimoxazole or sulphasalazine, which interfere with folic acid absorption and metabolism; and those with an increased demand engendered by haemoglobinopathy or multiple pregnancy. It is wise to give these patients folic acid, 5 mg daily, during pregnancy, to overcome any absorption defect, rather than rely on the small supplements in combined iron and folic acid preparations. The only risk is the possibility of treating a patient with undiagnosed true cyanocobalamin-dependent pernicious anaemia with folic acid alone. The chance of this has been estimated as 1 in 250 000 antenatal patients, and should be eliminated with a routine blood count.

It was shown convincingly by Hall (1972) that folic acid supplements, initiated at the first antenatal visit, had no effect on the catastrophes of late pregnancy such as antepartum haemorrhage. On the other hand, it is during the first trimester that the placenta is implanting and fetal need is greatest. Martin et al (1965) found an apparent benefit from folic acid supplements in patients with recurrent abortion. In 1980, after a study which took 12 years to complete, Smithells et al were able to show that in women who had had a fetus with a neural tube defect, supplementary vitamins and minerals, including folic acid, 0.36 mg/day, started at least 4 weeks before conception and continued until the time of the second missed period, reduced the recurrence rate from 5.0 per cent to 0.6 per cent. Laurence et al (1980) achieved a somewhat smaller reduction in recurrent neural tube defects from 7 per cent to 3 per cent, by preconceptional dietary counselling alone. In 1981 Laurence et al produced some evidence that the active component was folic acid. They gave 4 mg folic acid daily, starting from the time contraceptive precautions were stopped and continued through the first trimester. There were no recurrences amongst the 44 women complying, but 4 of the 51 women given placebo tablets had another baby with a neural tube defect.

It is possible that the effect of folic acid supplements initiated before conception may help to prevent congenital defects other than those of the neural tube. There is a case for seeing any woman who has had an abnormal baby for preconceptional counselling, performing a blood count and initiating folic acid supplements. There are some theoretical reasons for believing that folic acid may also influence early placental development, and it is my own practice to adopt the same manoeuvre with women who have lost a baby from placental insufficiency in association with essential hypertension, or from abruptio placentae.

*Teenagers*. The adolescent mother-to-be requires nutrition for her growth as well as the pregnancy. Individual dietary assessment and counselling is desirable (see Shervington 1974).

*Dietary fads*. Vegetarians and adherents of doctrinal dietary philosophies require individual assessment. Those who will eat cheese, eggs and fish and drink milk give rise to little difficulty; any need for iron supplements is reflected by haemoglobin estimations. When the patient will not eat animal protein in any form, specialist dietetic advice may be required to ensure an adequate intake of essential amino acids. Considerable ingenuity will also be required to provide adequate levels of minerals and vitamins if the patient also has a aversion to oral or parenteral medication. Reference to Paul and Southgate (1978) may be helpful in finding acceptable foods which will make up basic requirements.

*Asian women* living in Europe often have a low vitamin D intake and, because of their clothing and tendency to stay indoors, little exposure to sunlight. As a result, their vitamin D status in pregnancy is often borderline. Brooke et al (1981) showed that serum 25-hydroxy vitamin D levels are low during pregnancy, and particularly low postpartum and in the newborn of Asian women in London. This alone does not prove that they were adversely affected, as their calcitriol (1,25-dihydroxy vitamin D) levels may have been maintained, but alkaline phosphatase bone isoenzyme was elevated in 20 per cent of the patients postpartum, and 50 per cent of the newborn. This is suggestive of sub-clinical bone disease. Maxwell et al (1981) have found that giving British Asians vitamin D supplements, 25 μg (1000 i.u.) daily results in better maternal and newborn protein nutrition and less low-birth-weight babies. There is thus a case for giving a preparation like Calcium with Vitamin D tablets, B.N.F., two daily throughout pregnancy, to Asian women living in Europe.

*Underprivileged individuals*. The first consideration in dealing with undernourished pregnant women in impoverished circumstances or underdeveloped countries is to ensure adequate protein nutrition. The simplest basis is 1 litre of cow's milk or equivalent dried milk daily. This provides about 35 g protein, 38 g fat and 47 g carbohydrate, amounting to about 700 kcal (2940 kJ), and in addition 1.2 g calcium, 0.12 g magnesium, 0.95 g phosphorus and 5 mg of iron. Consideration of the diet the patient is receiving and supplementary vitamin and iron tablets makes it possible to make up acceptable nutrition.

## GENERAL AND HYGIENIC FACTORS

*Exercise, work and travel*. Obstetricians are sometimes required to pronounce on these. It is often best, having ascertained what the patient wants to do, to give firm confirmatory advice. This is necessary to counteract the comments of well-meaning relatives and friends, who otherwise may try to treat the antenatal patient as an invalid or, at the other extreme, encourage regular exercise when the patient wants to rest.

There are certain principles which help. The lethargy that is so common in early pregnancy is probably an effect of progesterone (Merryman et al 1954) or its metabolites (Holzbauer 1976). Some tolerance to the tiredness is acquired by mid-pregnancy, but in the last trimester the mechanical effects of increased body weight, changes in posture and abdominal distension again contribute to becoming tired easily. The patient's own reaction to these influences is the best guide, provided two problems are avoided. One is the psychological interpretation that pregnancy is an illness and the fetus is to blame for the mother's need to rest; or, alternatively, that these effects must be defeated by whatever activity the patient regards as normal. The other is a tendency to fill time whilst resting by consuming an excess of calories. As to exercise, vigorous equestrian activity has been blamed for premature rupture tof the membranes, and strenuous athletics are probably best avoided.

Some women find work a strain from the time they miss a period; others are psychologically and physically conditioned to working until the day they go into labour. It is best to agree with them. Travel is again a matter of common sense, but airline regulations should be taken into account. It has been suggested that the atmospheric pressure changes involved in air travel can predispose to premature rupture of the membranes. Whether or not this is true, an aeroplane is not the most propitious place to deliver a premature baby and patients at particular risk for this complication should avoid air travel between 26 and 34 weeks. In general the best service an obstetrician can perform for a pregnant woman intending to travel abroad is to provide her with the name and address of a reliable obstetrician or hospital in the area she is going to visit.

In patients with threatened abortion,Diddle et al (1953) showed that of 7981 women treated with partial bed rest, sedation and hormone supplements, 11.2 per cent proceeded to abortion. Of 793 women with threatened abortion who were instructed to resume their normal daily activities without any treatment at all, 8.1 per cent had an abortion. Sic!

*Clothing.* The only advice most pregnant women need is to put comfort before fashion for a few months. Both calf-and full length stockings with elastic tops should be avoided.

*Bathing and douching.* Attempts to convert British women from baths to showers and bidets, on the grounds that infection may occur, have been a dismal failure. In real life, bath water does not enter the vagina, unless a deliberate attempt is made to introduce it. Douching is contraindicated in pregnancy, as there is a risk of the douche fluid entering the uterus and of air embolus. The practice of douching is rare in Great Britain, but European and American women may need information on this point.

*Coitus*. Primigravid patients tend to show little sexual interest in the first trimester and they complain of breast tenderness during arousal (Masters and Johnson 1966). In the second trimester libido returns, but it is reduced again towards the end of pregnancy. There is no objective evidence that coitus causes abortion in a normal pregnancy and Pugh and Fernandez (1953) found that coitus in late pregnancy was not responsible for pregnancy complications. Unsolicited advice to avoid intercourse in pregnancy can cause marital disharmony, and lead to extramarital sexual activity (Masters and Johnson 1966).

On the other hand, the introduction of high concentrations of prostaglandins into the vagina at the times when the risk is greatest would seem unwise in women with threatened or habitual abortion, and in those at risk for premature labour. Goodlin (1969) found that orgasm is also associated with uterine contractions and premature labour sometimes starts in this way.

## VACCINATION AND IMMUNISATION

In general live vaccines are best avoided in pregnancy, even though the risk of infecting the conceptus may be very small. The hazards of toxin preparations or immune sera are simply those of pyrexial or other systemic reactions.

*Rubella*. There is no effective killed virus preparation and rubella vaccination should not be conducted during pregnancy. The potential disaster if an apparently harmless strain of virus used for immunisation that proved to be infective to the fetus would be so great that, although perhaps remote and theoretical, the risk is not worth taking. Puerperal immunisation, accompanied by contraception for three months, is appropriate for patients who are serum negative in pregnancy.

High-titre anti-rubella immunoglobulin should be reserved for serum negative patients and those taking immunosuppressive drugs, and given within a very few days of definite exposure to an infective case of rubella. It only conveys limited protection, and used more widely simply obscures the serological reactions of patients who were not actually at risk.

*Smallpox*. There is a risk of fatal fetal vaccinia if primary vaccination or revaccination after many years is carried out in pregnancy. The need should now be extremely rare; if it ever occurs, simultaneous administration of anti-vaccinal gamma globulin should confer some protection to the fetus.

*Poliomyelitis*. Live vaccines are used. The risk of poliomyelitis is now so small in developed countries that the theoretical and equally small risk that the attenuated virus might harm the fetus is not worth taking. In an epidemic situation the wild virus presents a much greater risk and pregnant women should then be immunised.

*Influenza*. Greenberg et al (1958) reviewed mortality in New York during the Asian influenza epidemic of 1957. Ten per cent of the deaths were in pregnant women and nearly half the women of reproductive age who died were pregnant. More recently, it has been demonstrated that maternal influenza in pregnancy is associated with an incidence of 3 to 4 per 1000 of leukaemia and related conditions in childhood, in the offspring (Fedrick and Alberman 1972). On the other hand the risk of maternal death from influenza is numerically minute, and though the association with childhood leukaemia has been confirmed in other studies, there is no convincing evidence that the relation is causal.

In an epidemic, it is therefore reasonable to immunise pregnant women against influenza, particularly if a killed virus preparation is available. If the procedure was employed more widely there is a chance that severe reactions, particularly in women with an allergic diathesis, might do more harm than the influenza.

*Hepatitis B*. Hepatitis B carriers represent between 0.1 and 0.6 per cent of the antenatal population in Great Britain (Derso et al 1978, Roddick 1983) and considerably more in the United States of America. The hazards they engender are principally blood-borne, and to their medical and nursing attendants. Vertical transmission to the baby is a risk in patients from the Far East (Woo et al 1979) who carry the $HB_e$ antigen, which probably signifies the presence of replicating virus and is an infectivity marker. The newborn babies of these women may benefit from administration of specific antihepatitis B immunoglobulin.

*Varicella*. Chicken pox and zoster are unusual in pregnancy but a very few cases of related fetal brain and limb damage have been reported. If a pregnant woman has been in contact with the disease and gives no history of the illness, a dose of zoster immune globulin given within three days may protect the fetus against infection. (Waterson 1979). The immune globulin should also be given to the newborn babies of women who have varicella within a few days of the confinement.

*Typhoid and paratyphoid A and B* vaccines are made from killed bacteria. Their only risk is of a pyrexial reaction.

*Tetanus, cholera and yellow fever* immunisations convey no known risk to the fetus.

## RADIATION AND ULTRASOUND

Evidence from retrospective studies and extrapolation from animal work, the effects of radiotherapy and the effects of exposure to the consequences of atomic explosions suggests that exposure to X-irradiation during pregnancy might be harmful to the fetus. The particular risks mentioned include death of the embryo, malformation of the fetus related to the gestation at the time of exposure, mental retardation and susceptibility to childhood malignant disease. Estimates of the dose of radiation necessary to place the fetus at risk vary widely. Brent (1967) and Sternberg (1973) concluded that the smallest dose that can be held to have a probable relationship to fetal abnormality is 50 rad (0.5 Gy) applied between the tenth and fortieth days after conception. Less than 25 rad (0.25 Gy) in protracted doses is held to bear an 'improbable relationship' to fetal abnormality. Mole (1979) considered that the excess risk of mental subnormality after exposure *in utero* to 5 rad (50 mGy) was less than 1 in 1000. In order to obtain some idea of how these figures relate to diagnostic X-rays in pregnancy, an abdominal X-ray in pregnancy involves fetal exposure to about 0.5 rad (5 mGy), a pelvimetry about 1.1 rad (11 mGy) (Ministry of Health 1960). It therefore seems that the ordinary use of diagnostic radiography in pregnancy carries no specifiable risk, though on general principles it should be kept to a minimum. Routine chest X-rays are scarcely justified when the diagnostic rate for tuberculosis is small. Where possible the fetus should be screened, the number of films taken (which may be considerably larger than the number sent to the clinician) should be strictly limited, and where reasonable, radiographic procedures should be postponed until the second trimester or the pregnancy is over.

Stewart and Kneale (1970) thought that abdominal X-rays in pregnancy were related to the incidence of childhood cancer in the offspring. Their studies were retrospective and based on comparisons with matched cases, and they did not take account of the possible effect of maternal age or the medical conditions for which the X-rays were performed. Their findings are in conflict with those of Court-Brown et al (1960) who found no increase in leukaemia in the children of 43 742 women who had abdominal or pelvic X-rays in pregnancy, including 553 who had intravenous urograms. There was no increase in leukaemia in the children exposed to radiation antenatally in Hiroshima and Nagasaki (Jablon and Kato 1970).

The 'ten day rule' employed by radiologists, confining X-rays to within 10 days of the last menstrual period to avoid irradiation of any early conceptus, is of dubious validity (Houston 1977, Mole 1979). At this time the conceptus is composed of totipotent cells, and would either be killed by a toxic effect or damaged cells would be replaced. There is no evidence of congenital abnormality arising from X-ray exposure arising at this time; or for that matter in the first half of the cycle, when the ovum is developing.

There is no evidence in humans of any second generation effect of diagnostic X-rays *in utero* on the reproductive performance of the offspring.

### Diagnostic ultrasonography

After suggestions that ultrasound examinations might cause chromosome aberrations, human lymphocyte cultures and also blood cell cultures from babies whose mothers had had ultrasound examinations during pregnancy have been examined by a number of authors. No convincing evidence of chromosome damage has been found. In clinical studies, Hellman et al (1970) found a fetal abnormality rate of 2.7 per cent in three countries which used ultrasound diagnostically, and considered this no greater than the general incidence in the populations studied. Nonetheless, it will take many years of follow-up of large series of patients before it will be possible to say with absolute confidence that ultrasound never does harm.

## DRUGS USED IN PREGNANCY

### Analgesics

Studies which claimed an association of the use of aspirin with congenital abnormalities were subject to biasing factors (Collins 1981), and the prospective Collaborative Perinatal Project (Slone et al 1976) found no evidence that the drug was a cause of fetal abnormality. Paracetamol (acetaminophen) is much more widely used in pregnancy and no harm has been suggested.

It is thought that aspirin and other salicylates, as prostaglandin synthesis inhibitors, may delay the spontaneous onset of labour and prolong its course if taken in full doses at the end of pregnancy (Lewis and Schulman 1973, Collins and Turner 1975). Of more significance is the suggestion that salicylates may impair platelet aggregation in newborn infants and predispose to intracranial haemorrhage in premature babies (Rumack et al 1981). Salicylates are probably best avoided by women prone to premature labour and by all women when the confinement is imminent.

The neonatal respiratory depression that can be the result of large doses of narcotic analgesics, including pethidine (meperidine), to relieve the pain of labour are well-known. Pain relief in labour is important and the drugs should not be withheld when they are needed. The use of preparations combining a morphine antagonist with pethidine has largely been abandoned. Their efficacy was always doubtful and it is simpler to provide effective newborn resuscitation should it be needed. If it is considered that a narcotic antagonist may be of value in the newborn, naloxone has the advantage over its predecessors that larger doses do not themselves produce respiratory depression.

Epidural analgesia with bupivacaine conveys no particular risk to the fetus provided maternal hypotension, which can cause fetal distress, is avoided. It is desirable to use preliminary fluid loading and monitor maternal blood pressure during the induction of the epidural block.

### Antacids

Nelson and Forfar (1971) found an apparent association between the use of antacids in the first eight weeks of pregnancy and congenital abnormalities of the fetus. There seemed to be no relation to any particular antacid and the association was not confirmed in the Royal College of General Practitioners' (1975) prospective study or other large surveys.

It is probably best to use Magnesium Trisilicate Mixture to treat dyspepsia in pregnancy when this is effective; Magnesium Hydroxide Mixture has the additional property of a mild laxative effect. There is no reason to believe that oxethazaine (Mucaine) or metoclopramide (Maxolon, Primperan) are harmful.

### Antiemetics

Nausea and vomiting in the second half of the first trimester may not justify hospital admission but can cause considerable misery to the pregnant woman. If the symptoms persist after iron tablets have been discontinued, urinary and other infections have been ruled out and simple measures such as biscuits first thing in the morning and then getting up very slowly, glucose sweets and small meals have failed, then the use of anti-emetics is contemplated. All the anti-emetics except promethazine have in turn been accused of teratogenicity and subsequently exonerated. The most recent target was Debendox (Bendectin), which contains dicyclomine, doxylamine and pyridoxine. Both the American courts and the Committee on Safety of Medicines (1981) in Great Britain have expressed themselves satisfied, on the basis of studies of many thousands of patients, that there is no evidence that the preparation is teratogenic in humans.

If anti-emetics are used, pyridoxine alone is worth a trial (American Medical Association Council in Pharmacy and Chemistry 1956). Metoclopramide, which has a central anti-emetic action and also promotes gastric emptying, is often effective (Sidhu and Lean 1970). Promethazine or its theoclate (Avomine) tend to make the patient sleepy but seem to be safe; Debendox may be reserved for problem cases. Last resorts include re-evaluation of diagnosis, hypnosis, trifluoperazine (Stelazine) or prochlorperazine (Stemetil) and steroids (Wells 1953).

## Diuretics

Finnerty and Bepko (1966) suggested the use of thiazide diuretics in young primigravidae for the prophylaxis of toxaemia. Their apparently favourable result is usually attributed to differences in the trial groups of patients. Menzies (1964) found chlorothiazide of more use than phenobarbitone and bed rest in managing mild preeclampsia, but this may have been due to a low grade antihypertensive effect of the drug. One of the babies died of neonatal thrombocytopenia purpura. The drugs can reduce plasma volume and contribute to intra-uterine growth retardation. (Campbell and MacGillivray 1975). Diuretics should be avoided during pregnancy unless needed to treat specific conditions such as heart disease.

## Laxatives

There is no indication that any of these preparations are teratogenic. It is possible that drastic purgation with colonic irritants can predispose to abortion by reflex stimulation of uterine contractions. Castor oil given at term, when it is not rejected by vomiting, results in a burst of colicky uterine contractions, sometimes accompanied by the signs of fetal distress. The mechanism is probably hydrolysis in the small intestine, followed by systemic absorption of ricinoleic acid, which is a potent myometrial stimulant.

Dietary measures and discontinuation of oral iron preparations if these are implicated are the first choice in treating constipation in pregnancy; bulk purgatives such as Magnesium Hydroxide Mixture are the second. Mineral oil preparations are best avoided. They are said to interfere with the absorption of fat soluble vitamins and to predispose to ano-rectal disorders. Of the irritant purgatives, preparations of senna seem to be the least drastic. More powerful irritants should be reserved for patients habituated to their use.

**Ovulation stimulants**

The incidence of multiple pregnancy when ovulation has been stimulated with clomiphene is about 7 per cent of twins and 0.9 per cent of greater multiples. There were 58 cases of major or minor fetal abnormality in 2369 pregnancies (2.4 per cent) in mothers treated with clomiphene (Merrell 1981) so there is no indication of any risk of teratogenesis in induced ovulation. On the other hand, eight of the abnormalities arose from 158 mothers who inadvertently received a course of clomiphene during the first six weeks after conception. If menstruation does not occur in a woman who has previously responded to clomiphene, then the results of a pregnancy test should be awaited before giving a further course.

Menotrophin (Pergonal) conveys a greater risk of multiple pregnancy, but does not appear to be teratogenic. Multiple pregnancies are less common when the dose of menotrophin is strictly controlled with daily oestrogen estimations.

There is good evidence (for example, see Griffith et al 1978) that bromocriptine is not teratogenic in humans. In general the drug is withdrawn after the first missed period or a positive pregnancy test, but consideration can be given to continuing its administration when there is evidence of a large pituitary tumour or expansion.

**Oxytoxic drugs**

The safety of intravenous oxytocin in reasonable doses for induction of labour and treatment of uterine inertia was proved as long ago as 1957, when Hellman et al accumulated the results from 5656 patients at 10 hospitals. The perinatal mortality in a group that must have been biased by high risk patients was 2.0 per cent; there were no maternal deaths and only one ruptured uterus—an incidence comparable to that associated with spontaneous labour. Alas, when the same drug is given in doses some 100 times greater by the buccal route, relying on a limited and erratic absorption process, hypertonic contracture of the uterus occurs in at least 1 per cent of cases and uterine rupture in about 1 in 500 patients.

Dihydrogenated ergot alkaloids and sparteine both appeared safe for induction of labour at first, when they were given to moderately sized series of normal patients. Only when these agents were employed in higher risk situations did their deleterious effects on perinatal mortality become apparent.

With prostaglandins used for the induction of labour, no series of cases of sufficient size to permit firm conclusions has yet been accumulated. Reports of rupture of the primigravid uterus associated with the employment of prostaglandin $E_2$ vaginal pessaries followed by epidural analgesia and oxytocin infusions (Scott and Lichter 1981, Geirsson 1981) give some cause for concern.

**Prostaglandin synthesis inhibitors**

This group of anti-inflammatory agents, which includes aspirin, fenoprofen, ibuprofen, indomethacin, ketoprofen, mefenamic acid and naproxen are not known to be teratogenic. On the other hand, given in late pregnancy they pass through to the fetus and may interfere with the prostaglandin $E_2$ mechanism which maintains patency of the fetal ductus arteriosus in the presence of a low blood $Po_2$. The consequences may be premature closure of the ductus with difficulty in establishing the pulmonary circulation at birth, or persistent pulmonary hypertension in the newborn (Rudolph 1981). It is inadvisable to use prostaglandin synthesis inhibitors in the attempt to suppress premature labour and best to find alternative remedies in the last few weeks of pregnancy for patients taking the drugs chronically.

**Sex hormones**

The subject of administration of sex hormones in pregnancy has recently been reviewed (Darling and Hawkins 1981).

*Oestrogens*. There is no established indication for the use of oestrogen supplements in pregnancy. Stilboestrol given in pregnancy led to minor vaginal structural and epithelial abnormalities (adenosis) and rare cases of vaginal adenocarcinoma in teenage female offspring, and possibly abnormalities of the genito-urinary tract in male offspring.

*Progestagens*. The only acceptable use for progestagen supplements in pregnancy is in women with recurrent abortion during the first trimester, if abnormally poor progesterone effects can be demonstrated in vaginal smears. Even then, the therapeutic value is doubtful and missed abortion may result. The progestagens which are known to be harmless are 17-hydroxy compounds; progesterone itself given as rectal suppositories and hydroxyprogesterone given intramuscularly, being the best examples. 19-*Nor*-steroids can, rarely, produce a transient enlargement of the clitoris in the female fetus and, more rarely, fusion of the labio-scrotal folds which requires incision.

*Oestrogen-progestagen combinations.* There was a very small risk of fetal abnormality, probably between 1 in 500 and 1 in 2000, affecting mainly male fetuses, if a woman became pregnant whilst taking a combined contraceptive pill. Whether or not this applies to current preparations with containing smaller doses of synthetic hormones is not clear. Nonetheless, pregnancy should be excluded before a patient starts taking the pill, and if a patient taking the pill unexpectedly misses a period, pregnancy should be excluded before she starts the next cycle of pills.

**Thyroxine**

In some environments it was the custom to give some women small doses of thyroxine in pregnancy on a flimsy pretext. These supplements appeared to do no harm.

REFERENCES

American Medical Association Council on Pharmacy and Chemistry 1956 Report of the Council. Current status of therapy in nausea and vomiting of pregnancy. Journal of the American Medical Association 160: 208–209

Bower D 1964 The influence of dietary salt intake on pre-eclampsia. Journal of Obstetrics and Gynaecology of the British Commonwealth 71: 123–125

Brent R L 1967 Medicolegal aspects of teratology. Journal of Pediatrics 71: 288–298

Brooke O G, Brown I R F, Cleeve H J W, Sood A 1981 Observations on the vitamin D state of pregnant Asian women in London. British Journal of Obstetrics and Gynaecology 88: 18–26

Bryce-Smith D, Waldron H A 1974 Lead in food—are today's regulations sufficient? Chemistry in Britain 10: 202–206

Bryce-Smith D, Stephens R 1981 Lead or health, 2nd edition. Conservation Society Pollution Working Party, London

Bryce-Smith D, Deshpande R R, Hughes J and Waldron H A 1977 Lead and cadmium levels in stillbirths. Lancet i: 1159

Campbell D M, MacGillivray I 1975 The effect of low-calorie diet or a thiazide on the incidence of pre-eclampsia and on birth weight. British Journal of Obstetrics and Gynaecology 82: 572–577

Carswell F, Kerr M M, Hutchison J H 1970 Congenital goitre and hypothyroidism produced by maternal ingestion of iodides. Lancet i: 1241–1243

Collins E 1981 Maternal and fetal effects of acetaminophen and salicylates in pregnancy. Obstetrics and Gynecology 58: 57–62

Collins E, Turner G 1975 Maternal effects of regular salicylate ingestion in pregnancy. Lancet ii: 335–338

Committee on Safety of Medicines 1981 Data sheet change—Debendox. Current Problems 6 (2)

Court-Brown W M, Doll R, Hill A B 1960 Incidence of leukaemia after exposure to diagnostic radiation in utero. British Medical Journal ii: 1539–1545

Darling M R, Hawkins D F 1981 Sex hormones in pregnancy. Clinics in Obstetrics and Gynaecology 8: 405–419

Department of Health and Social Security 1979 Recommended daily amounts of food, energy and nutrients for groups of people in the United Kingdom. Report by the Committee on Medical Aspects of Food Policy. DHSS Report on Health and Social Subjects 15

Derso A, Boxall E H, Tarlow M J, Flewett T H 1978 Transmission of $HB_sAg$ from mother to infant in four ethnic groups. British Medical Journal i: 949–952

de Snoo K 1937 The prevention of eclampsia. American Journal of Obstetrics and Gynecology 34: 911–939

Diddle A W, O'Connor K A, Jack R, Pearse R L 1953 Evaluation of bed rest in threatened abortion. Obstetrics and Gynecology 2: 63–67

Fedrick J, Alberman E D 1972 Reported influenza in pregnancy and subsequent cancer in the child. British Medical Journal ii: 485–488

Finnerty F A, Bepko F J 1966 Lowering the perinatal mortality and the prematurity rate: the value of prophylactic thiazides in juveniles. Journal of the American Medical Association 195: 429–432

Geirsson R T 1981 Uterine rupture following induction of labour with prostaglandin $E_2$ pessaries, an oxytocin infusion and epidural analgesia. Journal of Obstetrics and Gynaecology 2: 76–78

Gilfillan S C 1965 Lead poisoning and the fall of Rome. Journal of Occupational Medicine 7: 53–60

Goodlin R C 1969 Orgasm and premature labour. Lancet ii: 646

Greenberg M, Jacobziner H, Pakter J, Weisl B A G 1958 Maternal mortality in the epidemic of Asian influenza, New York City, 1957. American Journal of Obstetrics and Gynecology 76: 897–902

Griffith R W, Turkulj I, Braun P 1978 Outcome of pregnancy in mothers given bromocriptine. British Journal of Clinical Pharmacology 5: 227–231

Hall M H 1972 Folic acid deficiency and abruptio placentae. British Journal of Obstetrics and Gynaecology 79: 222–225

Hamlin R H J 1952 The prevention of eclampsia and pre-eclampsia. Lancet ii: 64–68

Hamlin R H J 1953 The prevention of pre-eclampsia by means of diet and weight control. Proceedings of the Royal Society of Medicine 46: 393–376

Hawkins D F 1981 Routine iron in pregnancy—is it necessary? Modern Medicine 26 (8): p 12

Heardman H 1959 Physiotherapy in obstetrics and gynaecology, 2nd edition. Livingstone, Edinburgh, p 65

Hellman L M, Duffus G M, Donald I, Sunden B 1970 Safety of diagnostic ultrasound in obstetrics. Lancet i: 1133–1134

Hellman L M, Kohl S G, Schechter H R 1957 Pitocin—1955. American Journal of Obstetrics and Gynecology 73: 507–517

Hemminki E, Starfield B 1978 Routine administration of iron and vitamins during pregnancy: review of controlled trials. British Journal of Obstetrics and Gynaecology 85: 404–410

Hillman R W, Cabaud P G, Schenone R A 1962 The effects of pyridoxine supplements on the dental caries experience of pregnant women. American Journal of Clinical Nutrition 10: 512–515

Holzbauer M 1976 Physiological aspects of steroids with anaesthetic properties. Medical Biology 54: 227–242

Houston C S 1977 Diagnostic irradiation of women during the reproductive period. Canadian Medical Association Journal 117: 648–651.

Jablon S, Kato H 1970 Childhood cancer in relation to prenatal exposure to atomic-bomb radiation. Lancet ii: 1000–1003.

Jewett J F, Reid D E, Safon L E ,Easterday G L 1968 Childbed fever—a continuing entity. Journal of the American Medical Association, 206: 344–350

Kelly A M, Macdonald D J, McNay M B 1977 Ferritin as an assessment of iron stores in normal pregnancy. British Journal of Obstetrics and Gynaecology 84: 434–438

Laurence K M, James N, Miller M, Campbell H 1980 Increased risk of recurrence of pregnancies complicated by fetal neural tube defects in mothers receiving poor diets, and possible effect of dietary counselling. British Medical Journal 281: 1592–1594

Laurence K M, James N, Miller M H, Tennant G B, Campbell H 1981 Double-blind randomised controlled trial of folate treatment before conception to prevent recurrence of neural-tube defects. British Medical Journal 282: 1509–1511

Leboyer F 1975 Birth without violence. Knopf, New York

Lewis R B, Schulman J D 1973 Influence of acetylsalicylic acid , an inhibitor of prostaglandin synthesis, on the duration of human gestation and labour. Lancet ii: 1159–1161

Lind T, Hytten F E, Thomson A M 1975 Anaemia in pregnancy. British Medical Journal i, 627

Lowe C R 1972 Congenital malformations and the problem of their control. British Medical Journal iii: 515–520

Martin R H, Harper T A, Kelso W 1965 Serum-folic-acid in recurrent abortions. Lancet i: 670–672

Masters W H, Johnson V A 1966 Human sexual response. Little, Brown, Boston

Maxwell J D, Ang L, Brooke O G, Brown I R F 1981 Vitamin D supplements enhance weight gain and nutritional status in pregnant Asians. British Journal of Obstetrics and Gynaecology 88: 987–991

Menzies D N 1964 Controlled trial of chlorothiazide in treatment of early pre-eclampsia. British Medical Journal i: 739–742

Merrell 1981 Clomid. In: Data sheet compendium 1981–82. Datapharm, London, pp 170–171

Merryman W, Borman R, Barnes L, Rothchild I 1954 Progesterone 'anaesthesia' in human subjects. Journal of Clinical Endocrinology and Metabolism 14. 1567–1569

Ministry of Health. Department of Health for Scotland 1960 Radiological hazards in patients. Second report of the Committee. Her Majesty's Stationery Office, London, p 934

Moghissi K S 1981 Risks and benefits of nutritional supplements during pregnancy. Obstetrics and Gynecology 58: 68–78S

Mole R H 1979 Radiation effects on pre-natal development and their radiological significance. British Journal of Radiology 52: 89–101

Morris M B, Weinstein L 1981 Caffeine and the fetus: is trouble brewing? American Journal of Obstetrics and Gynecology 140: 607–610

Moya F, Moroshima H O, Shnider S M, James L S 1965 Influence of maternal hyperventilation on the newborn infant. American Journal of Obstetrics and Gynecology 91: 76–88

Nelson M M, Forfar J O 1971 Associations between drugs administered during pregnancy and congenital abnormalities of the fetus. British Medical Journal i: 523–527

Nelson M N, Enkin M W, Saigal S, Bennett K J, Milner R, Sackett D L 1980 A randomized clinical trial of the Leboyer approach to childbirth. New England Journal of Medicine 302: 655–660

Niswander K R, Singer J, Westphal M, Weiss W 1969 Weight gain during pregnancy and prepregnancy weight. Association with birth weight of term gestation. Obstetrics and Gynaecology 33: 482–491

Nyirjesy L, Lonergan W M, Kane J J 1968 Clinical significance of total weight gain in pregnancy. Obstetrics and Gynecology 32: 391–396

Paul A A, Southgate D A T 1978 McCance and Widdowson's The composition of foods, 4th edition. Her Majesty's Stationery Office, London

Pugh W E, Fernandez F L 1953 Coitus in late pregnancy. A follow-up study. Obstetrics and Gynecology 2: 636–642

Robinson M 1958 Salt in pregnancy. Lancet i: 178–181

Roddick L G 1983 Obstetric patients with a serum hepatitis B surface antigen. Journal of Obstetrics and Gynaecology (in press)

Royal College of General Practitioners 1975 Morbidity and drugs in pregnancy. Journal of the Royal College of General Practitioners, 25: 631–645

Rudolph A M 1981 The effects of nonsteroidal anti-inflammatory compounds on fetal circulation and pulmonary function. Obstetrics and Gynecology 58: 63–67S

Rumack C M Guggenheim M A, Rumack B H, Peterson R G, Johnson M L, Braithwaite W R 1981 Neonatal intracranial hemorrhage and maternal use of aspirin. Obstetrics and Gynecology 58: 52–56S

Scott J M 1979 Prophylactic haematinics in pregnancy; should they be given? Intake (Abbott Laboratories Ltd) 66: 1 and 4

Scott J M, Govan A D T 1949 Anaemia of pregnancy in Glasgow and district. British Medical Journal ii: 1083–1087

Scott J W, Lichter M 1981 A case of primigravid uterine rupture. Journal of Obstetrics and Gynaecology 2: 74–75

Shervington P C (1974) Diet in pregnancy; hygiene; radiation effects; and the prophylaxis of virus infections. In: Hawkins D F (editor) Obstetric therapeutics. Baillière Tindall, London. pp 155–156

Sidhu M S, Lean T H 1970 The use of metoclopramide (Maxolon) in hyperemesis gravidarum. Proceedings of the Obstetrical and Gynaecological Society of Singapore 1: 43–46

Slone D, Heinonen O P, Kaufman D W, Siskind V, Monson R R, Shapiro S 1976 Aspirin and congenital malformations. Lancet i: 1173–1175

Smithells R W, Sheppard S, Schorah C J, Seller M J, Nevin N C, Harris R, Read A P, Fielding D W 1980 Possible prevention of neural-tube defects by periconceptional vitamin supplementation. Lancet i: 339–340

Sternberg J 1973 Radiation risk in pregnancy. Clinical Obstetrics and Gynecology 16: 235–278

Stewart R, Kneale G W 1970 Radiation dose effects in relation to obstetric X-rays and childhood cancers. Lancet i: 1185–1188

Taylor D J, Lind T 1976 Haematological changes during normal pregnancy: iron induced macrocytosis. British Journal of Obstetrics and Gynaecology 83: 760–767

Waterson A P 1979 Virus infections (other than rubella) during pregnancy. British Medical Journal ii: 564–566

Wells C N 1953 Treatment of hyperemesis gravidarum with cortisone. American Journal of Obstetrics and Gynecology 66: 598–601

Wilson J G 1973 Present status of drugs as teratogens in man. Teratology 7: 3–16

Woo D, Cummins M, Davies P A, Harvey D R, Hurley R, Waterson A P 1979 Vertical transmission of hepatitis B surface antigen in carrier mothers in two West London hospitals. Archives of Disease in Childhood 54: 670–675

# 7

*D. F. Hawkins*

# Drug treatment of medical disorders in pregnancy

A number of drugs which are used to treat medical disorders in pregnancy are known to convey a small hazard to the fetus. With nearly all of these agents careful therapeutics can minimise the risk.

**Anaesthetics**

In general, local anaesthesia in pregnancy creates no problems. The rare convulsive reaction to local anaesthetics could give rise to fetal anoxia if prompt attention was not paid to the patient's airway and there are experimental reasons for believing that anoxic episodes in the first trimester might interfere with fetal development (Robson et al 1965). It is preferable to defer non-urgent procedures to the second trimester, to pay careful attention to the maximum recommended doses of local anaesthetics, to beware inadvertent intravenous administration and to have resuscitative facilities available.

There have been reports of fetal bradycardia arising from paracervical blocks. These could have been due to interference with the pelvic nerve plexus affecting uterine blood flow or perhaps direct injection into the fetal scalp. The use of paracervical blocks has largely been abandoned. Prilocaine used for regional anaesthesia was reported to have caused fetal methaemoglobinaemia. Other agents such as bupivacaine used for epidural anaesthesia are not a hazard to the baby if maternal hypotension is prevented, and improve placental blood flow in patients with pre-eclampsia (Joupilla et al 1982). Pre-loading with a fluid infusion and frequent monitoring of maternal blood pressure and the fetal heart during induction of an epidural block are important in this respect.

General anaesthesia *per se* conveys no hazard to the fetus, though postponement of non-urgent procedures and avoidance of anoxia during necessary anaesthetics should be considered. With screening for sickle cell trait, normal anaesthetic competence, pre-oxygenation, cricoid pressure during intubation and good control of respiration, there is no real problem. In a recent survey of surgical procedures during pregnancy (Brodsky et al 1980) there was a small increase in abortions, attributable to the surgical assaults and the conditions for which they were undertaken, but no increase in congenital abnormalities. Unnecessarily large doses of short acting barbiturates for the induction of anaesthesia for caesarean section should be avoided, as this can contribute to neonatal asphyxia. Attention to lateral tilt of the patient to prevent supine hypotension and an optimum induction-delivery interval are important (Holdcroft et al 1974, Adeleye 1981).

There is current interest in the possible ill-effects of anaesthetic gases on pregnant operating theatre personnel. The evidence is circumstantial, being derived from animal experiments (Smith 1974, and see Vessey and Nunn 1980), from epidemiological surveys (see Vessey and Nunn 1980) and from retrospective surveys suggesting that exposure to volatile solvents used in industry may contribute to congenital abnormalities (see, for example, Holmberg 1979). The epidemiological studies have major defects, but it is possible to deduce from them that pregnant women working in operating theatres have an increased risk of abortion; there is no clear evidence that congenital abnormalities are increased by this occupation (Vessey and Nunn 1980). In addition it seems clear that female anaesthetists who do not work in pregnancy—and for that matter, the wives of male anaesthetists—have a slightly increased risk of abortion and probably of babies with congenital abnormalities. This suggests that any hazard may be related not only to the stresses to which they are subjected at work but also to inherent factors. It is wise to advise a less stressful occupation if pregnancy is planned (Hawkins and Love 1978, Vessey and Nunn 1980). The reduction of anaesthetic gas pollution in operating theatres by scavenging systems should be instituted as a matter of general principle, without the implication that harm has been demonstrated.

**Anticholinesterases**

Myasthenia gravis is a rare complication of pregnancy. Interaction with other drugs such as aminoglycoside antibiotics, and with ether or muscle relaxants in general anaesthesia, may all add to the neuromuscular blocking effect. Magnesium should not be used to treat pre-eclampsia; hypermagnesaemia can be dangerous in these patients. Procaine, which is normally hydrolysed by cholinesterase, should be avoided; lignocaine and bupivacaine are metabolised differently and are safe (de Swiet 1979). A situation where the mother has had an unduly large dose of anticholinesterase at the time of delivery can give rise to neuromuscular depression in the newborn.

**Anticoagulants**

For a number of years, phenindione was widely used in Great Britain to treat thrombosis and embolism in pregnancy, and for prophylaxis in appropriate patients. In general the drug was discontinued before labour was induced electively. If labour began spontaneously with the patient still anticoagulated, little harm seemed to result, whether or not vitamin K was given, provided the third stage was managed with scrupulous care. Regrettably, this use remained undocumented, partly because each unit only had a very few cases each year, and partly because little trouble seemed to arise. In recent years there have been a number of reports on the dire consequences of anticoagulant treatment during pregnancy (Villasanta 1965, Hirsh et al 1970, Hall et al 1980), including fetal abnormality, abortion, prematurity and stillbirth. It is curious how many of these reports have come from America. Certainly the fetal loss rates of 10 of 30 per cent reported from that continent are foreign to British experience.

The reasons for the pessimistic reports probably include the widespread use of bishydroxycoumarin (Dicumarol) in America in the past. This is a very slow-acting agent with marked cumulative properties, and levels of anticoagulation tend to drift slowly and unpredictably. The change in general preference from phenindione to warfarin, which is much shorter-acting and needs close control, may also be a factor. It has only recently been realised that 'loading' doses of this drug are both unnecessary and undesirable. The high levels of anticoagulation necessary in patients with plastic heart valves convey an added risk; comparably high levels may have been sought in patients who do not need them. The recognition of 'warfarin embryopathy' if the drug is used in the first trimester is an adverse factor in the statistics which should be avoidable.

Whilst the incidence of fetal abnormality with warfarin used in the first trimester is not clear and may be quite small, there is a definite risk, particularly when the drug is given between 6 and 9 weeks of pregnancy (Hall et al 1980). The consistent feature is nasal hypoplasia with the bridge of the nose depressed, but damage to bony epiphyses in a wide variety of sites occurs and there is a proportion of eye defects and other systemic abnormalities. A few babies whose mothers had warfarin started in the first trimester and continued throughout pregnancy exhibited mental retardation. Finally, a number of cases of central nervous system abnormalities have been found, some associated with obvious haemorrhage.

The first step in solving this problem is to persuade cardiac surgeons to use biological valves, which do not in general need maintenance anticoagulation, instead of plastic valves in women of reproductive age, regardless of the expense. The next is to review women who are at high risk for thrombosis or embolism before conception and consider if treatment of varicose veins, screening for and treatment of hypercoagulable states, and operative procedures to prevent pulmonary embolus might be of value. The significant risk of maternal death with antenatal pulmonary embolism (Department of Health and Social Security 1979) should be borne in mind. In the few patients where prophylactic anticoagulation is really necessary in the first trimester, the change to heparin must be made as soon as pregnancy is suspected. Subcutaneous heparin will usually be appropriate, but in the rare case where full anticoagulation is necessary, and in the acute situation, the only rational mode of administration is continuous intravenous infusion. Any form of intermittent injection gives oscillating blood levels which are of limited value and may be dangerous. Control of heparin treatment should be with clotting times; partial thromboplastin time estimations are too insensitive to the moderate levels required and heparin blood levels are unpredictably unreliable in a few patients. To adjust the clotting time of 0.5 ml of blood in a small clean test tube, shaken every 5 minutes at room temperature to between 20 and 30 minutes does not require sophisticated laboratory facilities. Pregnancy is rare in haemodialysis patients; when it does occur, reduced dialysis times and small volume disposable kidneys permit minimal heparinisation.

When a leg vein thrombosis occurs in pregnancy, there is little doubt that anticoagulation, initially with heparin, is indicated. In one review (Ullery 1954) maternal mortality due to pulmonary embolism after untreated leg vein thrombosis was 15 per cent. Out of 38 patients treated with anticoagulants, 7 had pulmonary emboli but none died. 'Superficial' venous thrombosis nearly always has an extension into the deep veins.

When maintained anticoagulation is necessary in the second and most of the third trimester, the closely controlled use of warfarin in reasonable. Plastic heart valve patients sometimes need full anticoagulation, and control must then be even closer. With the majority of patients 'thrombotest' times of between 9 and 15 per cent or prothrombin times about double the control are adequate and safer than attempting higher levels of anticoagulation.

If labour begins unexpectedly the level of anticoagulation is checked immediately. Should it be in the lower range (thrombotest above 9 per cent) there is no real need to take any action; sudden restoration of normal or hyper-coagulability at a high risk time can do more harm than good. If the level of anticoagulation is high (thrombotest below 9 per cent), then administration of a small dose of phytomenadione (5 mg slowly i.v., repeated in 3 hours if necessary) is reasonable, though it is unlikely to affect anticoagulant levels in the fetus (Larson et al 1978). Scalp electrodes are avoided and the usual doses of vitamin K are given to the baby at birth. Ideally treatment is changed to subcutaneous or intravenous heparin two weeks before the end of pregnancy, to allow the fetus time to generate sufficient vitamin K. An alternative is to make the change to heparin 3 days before elective induction of labour and give the fetus an intramuscular injection of vitamin K *in utero* (Larsen et al 1978). Heparin administration is discontinued when labour is induced and recommenced when the third stage is complete.

**Anticonvulsants**

There is little doubt that anticonvulsant drugs, including carbamazepine and phenobarbitone in anticonvulsant doses, have a mild teratogenic effect. Smithells (1976) reviewed the literature and estimated that the incidence of major malformations in babies whose epileptic mothers had received anticonvulsants during pregnancy was 6.0 per cent, compared with 1.4 per cent with epileptic mothers not on treatment. It might be thought that it is the epilepsy rather than the drugs which is the adverse factor, as it is the more severe epileptics that are under treatment in pregnancy. This is an unlikely explanation. The anticonvulsants are teratogenic in large doses in animals. They interfere with folate absorption and metabolism in humans and low plasma folate levels and even megaloblastic anaemia are found in unsupplemented pregnant women taking the drugs. Finally, although the spectrum of fetal abnormality found is wide, specific syndromes such as the fetal hydantoin syndrome (Hanson et al 1976) and that related to trimethadione (Feldman et al 1977) have been observed.

It is probable that the hazard of maternal anticonvulsant treatment to the fetus can be reduced to a minimum. Pre-conceptional counselling of epileptics is of great importance. Review of patients at this stage will reveal a proportion who have been taking drugs for 10 or 20 years without any fits, sometimes because they had a fit with a high pyrexia or some other illness many years before, and many more who are taking unnecessarily large doses. Folic acid supplements of the order of 5 mg daily must be instituted before conception if they are to prevent abnormalities which may be initiated in the first trimester. It has been claimed (Reynolds 1967) that folic acid can increase fit frequencies in some epileptics, but this is not general experience. In any event, if the folic acid supplements are started before pregnancy there is opportunity to adjust anticonvulsant doses appropriately. Finally, an improved prognosis may be often obtained by altering the drug regimen. The literature on this point is complex and conflicting (see, for example, Starreveld-Zimmerman et al 1974, and Speidel and Meadow 1972). In general it seems that combinations of drugs give a higher risk than single agents. This could be related to competition of anticonvulsants for binding sites on plasma albumin (Monks et al 1978) resulting in higher free plasma levels of one or other of the drugs. Carbamazepine and phenobarbitone may be more benign than the other agents, if fits can be controlled adequately using one of these drugs alone.

During pregnancy, no attempt should be made to maintain 'normal therapeutic levels' in the plasma. Total plasma anticonvulsant levels fall due to impaired absorption and increased metabolism, but albumin binding is decreased (Perucca et al 1981), and the level of free drug may be adequate to control fits. If monitoring is desirable, either free plasma levels or salivary levels, which reflect them, are the appropriate measure in pregnancy. If fits occur during pregnancy, prompt treatment to clear the airway and obtain control with intravenous diazepam or chlormethiazole must be instituted to avoid fetal anoxia.

Treatment with anticonvulsants can produce a coagulation defect in the fetus which can be corrected with vitamin K. Phytomenadione should be given to the mother intravenously at the onset of labour, and to the newborn after delivery. Babies of mothers on anticonvulsants may suffer from a newborn withdrawal syndrome (Desmond et al 1972, Cree et al 1973). They should be observed for hypotonia, hypothermia and apnoeic attacks for two days after birth.

**Antidepressants and tranquillisers**

Pre-conceptional counselling is of value with all patients taking psychotropic drugs. As a matter of general principle, drug therapy can be reviewed and perhaps reduced; the drugs given can be changed from the latest psychotropic agents whose possible effects on the fetus are ill-documented to well tried remedies which have been used in pregnancy for many years. More important is recognition of the opportunity to wean the patient off drugs entirely and institute psychotherapeutic management. In pregnancy the door is wide open for this approach (Goldie 1974). Not only is there a major role change in progress, but also the reinforcement that drugs may harm the baby.

*Phenothiazines*. There is no clear evidence that these drugs are teratogenic; if there is any risk, it is very small (Beeley 1981). On the other hand the drugs are best not continued for more than a week or two, particularly in late pregnancy; isolated cases of extrapyramidal reactions in neonates have been reported (Levy and Wisniewsky 1974).

*Meprobamate.* No causal relationships of this drug to fetal abnormality has been established, though there are a few anecdotal reports of associations. Milkovich and van den Berg (1974) found 5 cases of congenital heart disease in the babies of 66 mothers who had received meprobamate during the first 6 weeks of pregnancy. When a larger series of cases was examined by Hartz et al (1975) there was no evidence of a teratogenic effect.

*Amine oxidase inhibitors.* There is no evidence that these agents are teratogenic. The reasons for avoiding their use in pregnancy are those associated with the use of β-sympathomimetics or of emergency general anaesthesia when the doctors concerned are unaware that the patient is taking the drug.

*Tricyclic antidepressants.* These have been reviewed by Nishimura and Tanimura (1976b), who concluded that there is no evidence of a causal relationship to fetal abnormality in humans. There is a chance that they might potentiate the effects of β-sympathomimetics. Tricyclics are slowly metabolised by the fetus and there are isolated reports of sympathomimetic and parasympatholytic effects in the newborn of mothers who have been taking the drugs in late pregnancy.

*Lithium.* The evidence on lithium is not conclusive, being based in part on selective and retrospective reports, but an undue proportion of congenital cardiovascular abnormalities are associated with administration in the first trimester (Schou et al 1973a, Weinstein 1976). Its use should be discontinued in patients planning pregnancy, and all women on lithium treatment should be warned to cease taking it immediately if they suspect they might be pregnant. Major cardiovascular anomalies arise between 5 and 9 weeks after the last menstrual period in humans. (Nishimura and Tanimura 1976a).

Close monitoring of serum levels, preferably to below 1.0 mmol/l, is needed if lithium treatment is used in late pregnancy and sodium depletion and diuretics avoided. Excess lithium can produce hypotonia and cyanosis in the newborn and thyroid function should be assessed in the newborn as there is a suspicion it may be affected. The mother's lithium clearance falls abruptly in the puerperium (Schou et al 1973b) and estimations of serum levels are necessary if toxicity is to be avoided.

### Antithyroid drugs

Pre-conceptional assessment should include selection of some patients for partial thyroidectomy. Those needing large doses of antithyroid drugs, those who find it difficult to comply with treatment regimens, those with bulky goitres and those with goitres extending near to the thoracic inlet are appropriate candidates. The other objective should be to secure euthyroidism at the time of conception. Myxoedema is associated with spontaneous abortion (Man et al 1951) and uncontrolled thyrotoxicosis with maternal and fetal morbidity and mortality (Gardiner-Hill 1929). Patients who want to breast feed babies should be managed on propylthiouracil, of which only small amounts appear in breast milk (Kampmann et al 1980); breast feeding is contraindicated if the mother is taking carbimazole.

The hazards of well controlled treatment with antithyroid drugs such as carbimazole or propylthiouracil in pregnancy are not great (Chahal et al 1981). There is a tendency to intra-uterine growth retardation, but the babies subsequently develop normally (Burrow et al 1968, McCarrol et al 1976). The newborn are examined for goitre, for neonatal hypothyroidism induced by transplacental passage of antithyroid drugs and for hyperthyroidism, which is occasionally caused by persistence of thyroid-stimulating immunoglobulins of maternal origin. With good management, these problems affect only about 3 per cent of the newborn.

In recent years it has been argued that combined treatment with antithyroid drugs and thyroxine is illogical, since thyroxine crosses the placenta so slowly (Fisher et al 1977). Nonetheless, the incidence of fetal loss seems to be reduced with a combined regimen (Chahal et al 1981). This may be due to damping of the untoward effects of poorly controlled administration of antithyroid drugs, and combined treatment should be considered when biochemical facilities are limited or patient compliance suspect. When partial thyroidectomy is indicated in pregnancy by enlargement or nodular change in the goitre or by inability of the patient to take drugs correctly, the middle trimester is the best time for the operation and the patients do well.

Iodine and medicines containing this element are contraindicated in pregnancy. The iodine is concentrated in the fetal thyroid gland and may produce fetal goitre and hypothyroidism (Carswell et al 1970).

### Cytotoxic drugs

Until recently, knowledge of the ill-effects of these drugs in human pregnancy has been scanty, but a number of women under treatment for malignant conditions have now had successful pregnancies. The reviews by Sweet and Kinzie (1976) and Barber (1981) are informative. Sweet and Kinzie record 164 women who had antineoplastic drugs in the first trimester, of whom 19 produced abnormal babies. In patients given cytotoxic drugs in the second and third trimesters, there was not a single fetal abnormality in 76 pregnancies.

Of the alkylating agents, a few women who had nitrogen mustard in the first trimester had normal babies, though fetal abnormalities have been recorded with cyclophosphamide and chlorambucil. With busulphan, 20 out of 22 women had normal babies. Antimetabolites seem to be more dangerous. Many patients have an abortion if the folic acid antagonists such as aminopterin or methotrexate are used in the first trimester, and up to half of the surviving pregnancies may result in an abnormal baby. On the other hand a number of women have had successful pregnancies after the use of mercaptopurine in the first few weeks. There is too little information on other agents such as actinomycin, cytarabine, fluorouracil, hydroxyurea, urethane, and vinca alkaloids in humans to form an opinion, but they are all teratogenic in animals. It is usually said that combinations of drugs are more hazardous than a single agent, but the evidence is obscure.

It therefore seems that the woman with leukaemia or a related disorder who wishes to have a baby, knowing the risks, should preferably wait until she is in remission or can be controlled by leucophoresis in the first trimester. Otherwise attempts should be made to control the disease with an appropriate agent used alone during the first few weeks.

Local applications of cytotoxic drugs, such as podophylline for warts or idoxuridine for *herpesvirus hominis* infections have been claimed to be responsible for anecdotal cases of congenital malformation. The evidence is obscure, but alternative methods of treatment are preferable in pregnancy.

**Diuretics**

Thiazide diuretics are best avoided in pregnancy unless there is a firm indication for their use. Chlorothiazide itself probably has a low grade antihypertensive action in some women but may reduce plasma volume and its use has been associated with reduced birth weight (Campbell and MacGillivray 1975). Plasma potassium levels may fall; oral potassium supplements have little effect on this. The mild hypokalaemia is not harmful unless exacerbated by ptyalism or vomiting. Two fatal cases of neonatal thrombocytopenia have been reported after the use of chlorothiazide (Menzies 1964, Rodriguez et al 1974) but this must be extremely rare, as the drug was widely used in pregnancy in the 1960s. There is a case for using chlorothiazide to treat carpal tunnel syndrome or gross oedema causing discomfort. The idea that the drug 'masks' the signs of developing pre-eclampsia is as fallacious in practice as the idea that aspirin masks a pyrexial illness.

Frusemide is a much more potent agent and conveys a real risk if reducing intravascular volume and placental perfusion, especially when there is already haemoconcentration due to pre-eclampsia (Liley 1970). The drug is sometimes valuable to prevent plasma expansion and left ventricular failure during blood or plasma expanding infusions. Continued use in pregnancy should be restricted to patients with heart or renal disease where it is considered essential—and it was a sad day for obstetricians when fashion swung from digitalis to frusemide in the management of heart failure. Patients taking frusemide should be monitored for a rising haematocrit and the development of postural hypotension as signs that reduced intravascular volume is becoming a serious problem, placing the fetus at risk unless the dose is reduced. Plasma expansion with albumin or other infusions is undertaken, or the baby is delivered.

## Hypoglycaemic drugs

Patients with diabetes mellitus should be reviewed before conception, with the object of establishing good control from the start of the first trimester. Measurement of haemoglobin $A_1$ offers a prospect of assessing the adequacy of recent treatment. The increased incidence of congenital abnormality in diabetes is known to be related to poor control, and it seems likely that the residual incidence of abnormalities is due to failure to establish rigid blood sugar control from conception onwards.

There is no convincing evidence that oral hypoglycaemic agents are teratogenic, but most physicians feel that better results are obtainable with insulin in pregnant diabetics not controlled with diet alone (de Swiet 1979). If chlorpropamide is used, hypoglycaemia may persist in the newborn (Zucker and Simon 1968).

## Hypotensive drugs

Obstetricians on both sides of the Atlantic show a clear preference for the use of methyldopa in treating essential hypertension in pregnancy (Lewis et al 1980). Apart from protecting the mother, methyldopa is the only hypotensive agent which has been clearly demonstrated to improve fetal prognosis (Leather et al 1968).

Redman et al (1976) had only 1 perinatal death in 117 patients treated with this drug. Postural hypotension and depression do not seem to be such prominent features of methyldopa treatment in pregnancy as they are in the non-pregnant patient. Occasionally the newborn will have a positive Coombs test but methyldopa haemolytic anaemia has not been reported in the newborn. A few cases of meconium ileus have occurred in the newborn of patients receiving 2 g or more of methyldopa daily (Clark et al 1972).

Hydralazine is a very useful drug to supplement methyldopa treatment over two or three weeks, when control of blood pressure with the latter drug alone becomes difficult. Used for a longer time hydralazine causes troublesome side effects, with skin rashes, headaches, nausea and tachycardia. It has been shown to improve at least myometrial blood flow (Johnson and Clayton 1957). There is no significant evidence of teratogenicity in humans, but a very small increase in birth defects in patients treated with the drug in one study (Heinonen et al 1977) suggests that it may better be avoided in the first trimester. The difference between the oral dose of 25 to 50 mg and the parenteral dose of 5 to 15 mg should be noted.

Opinions on the use of β-sympatholytic drugs in pregnancy vary from the idea that they are entirely benign (Eliahou et al 1978) to the view that their use is associated with something like a 50 per cent perinatal mortality (Stirrat and Lieberman 1977). The latter outcome has been said to be due to reduction of maternal cardiac output, prevention of vasodilatation in the placental blood supply, impairment of autonomic reflexes in the newborn and neonatal respiratory depression. The answer to this conflict of views seems to be that the β-blockers are relatively harmless to the fetus if initiated before the pregnancy begins and used in the small or moderate doses used to treat arrhythmias, hypertrophic cardiomyopathy or mild hypertension. It is when the drugs are employed in full doses in mid or late pregnancy to treat severe hypertension, perhaps out of control with other agents, that the fetal prognosis is poor. In these circumstances it is difficult to differentiate the consequences of the drugs from those of the hypertensive disease.

In general the treatment of pre-eclampsia which is becoming a hazard to mother or baby is to deliver the baby. In patients with an onset of hypertension between 28 and 32 weeks it may be advantageous to institute treatment. Gallery et al (1979) had a mixed series of patients, but it is possible to deduce that oxprenolol used at this stage at least does no harm to the fetus, while protecting the mother.

The use of ganglion-blockers in pregnancy resulted in a 50 per cent fetal loss associated with newborn hypotension and paralytic ileus (Morris 1953). Protoveratrine was used to control severe hypertension in mid or late pregnancy; its effect depended on the Bezold-Jarisch reflex, arising from receptors in the heart itself, and causing bradycardia and peripheral vasodilatation. Even when the drug was given by intravenous infusion, control was erratic; fetal prognosis was not improved (Carey 1959). Reserpine required a steadily increasing dose to maintain control, to a point where the mother could become autonomically denervated; it also caused newborn nasal obstruction, lethargy and sometimes hypothermia, and should not be used in pregnancy. Guanethidine is a useful oral agent, but should be discontinued 3 or 4 weeks before delivery to allow recovery of maternal autonomic function.

Too little is known about the modes of action or effects of clonidine or debrisoquine in pregnancy to be confident of their safety. Efforts have been made recently to popularise the α- and β-blocker labetalol in pregnancy, but the consistency of response is not such as to encourage its use in severe hypertension. The α-blocker prazosin has been used in small series of patients with apparent safety, but the unpredictability of response and consequent need to start with a very small dose and repeated increments render it unsuitable for dealing with severe hypertension.

Diazoxide produces a dramatic fall in blood pressure which may persist for days when given as a bolus dose intravenously. The suddenness of the response and the unpredictability of the response to the first dose do not encourage its use in pregnancy. Chronic administration is undesirable because of maternal hyperglycaemia and of inhibition of uterine contractions in labour; with large doses the neonate may have alopecia (Milner and Chouksey 1972) and neonatal glucose tolerance may be impaired.

**Immunosuppressives**

The subject of corticosteroids has been dealt with elsewhere (Chapter 10). Perhaps the insignificance of any risk of teratogenesis with steroids is best summed up by saying that after their use on many thousands of pregnant women over 25 years, it is still not possible to state if there is a very small risk of cleft palate or not.

That the combination of azathioprine with steroids is not teratogenic can be deduced from the data on patients with renal transplants who have gone through pregnancy taking these drugs. Rudolph et al (1979) reviewed continuing pregnancies in these patients. The incidence of spontaneous abortion (8.7 per cent), ectopic gestation (0.6 per cent) and stillbirth (1.9 per cent) did not differ significantly from those in a normal pregnant population.

Urinary tract infections, proteinuria, hypertension and pre-eclampsia were common, as might be expected in patients with a renal problem. Forty-four per cent of the live babies were of low birth weight (<2500 g). The pregnancies resulted in 221 term and 55 premature babies and 4 sets of twins. The incidence of congenital abnormalities was not increased. There were 10 neonatal deaths, eight from complications of prematurity, one from sepsis and one with a diaphragmatic hernia. The majority of the babies were known to be alive and well, the eldest being 10 years of age at the time of the report. The European Dialysis and Transplant Association (1980) found essentially similar results in their series. The incidence of multiple births was a little high; 97 transplant patients gave birth to 110 babies including 4 pairs of twins and 1 set of triplets. Among the babies, one had plagiocephaly with neurological damage, one mild mitral regurgitation, one pes equinovarus and one hypospadias.

It therefore seems that immunosuppressive dosee of azathioprine cannot be considered teratogenic in humans. The complications of pregnancy and the consequences to the fetus are simply those of renal disease. The combination of steroids and azathioprine may render the mother and the fetus more susceptible to infections.

Sulphasalazine is used in the treatment of inflammatory bowel conditions such as Crohn's disease and ulcerative colitis. The drug inhibits absorption of folates (Halstead et al 1981) and patients with these conditions should have folic acid supplements initiated before conception and continued throughout the pregnancy.

**Radiochemicals**

Iodine is concentrated in the fetal thyroid gland throughout the second and third trimesters and radioactive isotopes given to the mother can damage the fetal thyroid (Nishimura and Tanimura 1976c). Radioactive $^{131}$I should not be used for thyroid function testing or scanning the gland during pregnancy. $^{125}$I has a shorter half-life but $^{125}$I-labelled fibrinogen detection of deep vein thrombosis should also be avoided during pregnancy. Alternative methods are available for testing thyroid function; a thyroid nodule developing in pregnancy can be scanned using pertechnate with a very small exposure to radioactivity; surgical exploration may be preferred. The diagnosis of deep vein thrombosis in pregnancy is primarily clinical. If proof of the extent of the lesion is considered necessary, X-ray venography is possible.

Radioactive $^{32}$P should be avoided as it is teratogenic in animals and venesection is a preferable treatment if polycythaemia is diagnosed in pregnancy.

Radioactive xenon, $^{133}Xe$, is sometimes used by inhalation to estimate uterine blood flow in pregnancy. The exposure of the fetus to radiation is minutely small, of the order of 3 mrad (30 $\mu$Gy) (Jacoby et al 1972).

### Tropical diseases

With nearly all tropical diseases, effective remedies are available which can be used without significant risk to the fetus. We have recently reviewed this subject (Ledward and Hawkins 1982).

### Vitamin D

It has been suggested that large doses of vitamin D in pregnancy can be responsible for a syndrome of cranio-facial abnormalities and aortic stenosis, together with neonatal hypercalcaemia, but the syndrome occurs without vitamin D treatment (Antia et al 1967). Goodenday and Gordan (1971) found that doses of vitamin D used to maintain normal calcium and phosphate levels in women with hyperparathyroidism in pregnancy had no adverse effects on the babies.

Nonetheless, it is wise to restrict the dose to 25 $\mu$g (1000 iu) daily if vitamin D supplements are given to healthy women, and to control doses in patients having vitamin D treatment for calcium disorders with frequent plasma calcium and phosphate estimations.

## CONCLUSION

The manoeuvre which shows the greatest potential for further reduction of the small excess of fetal abnormalities associated with drugs used to treat medical conditions during pregnancy is pre-conceptional review of such patients and their treatment.

## REFERENCES

Adeleye J A 1981 The induction-delivery interval and fetal depression at caesarean section. Journal of Obstetrics and Gynaecology 2: 29–31

Antia A U, Wiltse H E, Rowe R D, Pitt E L, Levin S, Ottesen O E, Cooke R E 1967 Pathogenesis of the supravalvular aortic stenosis syndrome. Journal of Pediatrics 71: 431–441

Barber H R K 1981 Fetal and neonatal effects of cytotoxic agents. Obstetrics and Gynecology 58: 41S–47S

Beeley L 1981 Adverse effects of drugs in the first trimester of pregnancy. Clinics in Obstetrics and Gynaecology 8: 261–274

Brodsky J B, Cohen G J, Brown B W Jr, Wu M L, Whitcher C 1980 Surgery during pregnancy and fetal outcome. American Journal of Obstetrics and Gynecology 138: 1165–1167

Burrow G N, Burtsocas C, Klatskin E H, Grunt J A 1980 Children exposed *in utero* to propylthiouracil; subsequent intellectual and physical development. American Journal of Diseases in Childhood 116: 161–165

Campbell D M, MacGillivray I 1975 The effect of a low calorie diet or a thiazide diuretic on the incidence of pre-eclampsia and on birth weight. British Journal of Obstetrics and Gynaecology 82: 572–577

Carey H M 1959 Protoveratrine in the treatment of hypertension during pregnancy. New Zealand Medical Journal 58: 467–479

Carswell F, Kerr M M, Hutchison J H 1970 Congenital goitre and hypothyroidism produced by maternal ingestion of iodides. Lancet i: 1241–1243

Chahal P, Sidhu R, Joplin G F, Hawkins D F 1981 Treatment of thyrotoxicosis in pregnancy. Journal of Obstetrics and Gynaecology 2: 11–19

Clark A D, Sevitt L H, Hawkins D F 1977 Use of frusemide in severe toxaemia of pregnancy. Lancet i: 35–36

Cree J E, Meyer R, Hailey J M 1973 Diazepam in labour: its metabolism and effect on the clinical condition and thermogenesis of the newborn. British Medical Journal iv: 251–255

Department of Health and Social Security 1979 Report on confidential enquiries into maternal deaths in England and Wales 1973–1975 Report on Health and Social Subjects 14. Her Majesty's Stationary Office, London

Desmond M M, Schwaneke R P, Wilson G S, Yasunaga S, Burgdoff J 1972 Maternal barbiturate utilization and neonatal withdrawal symptomatology. Journal of Pediatrics 80: 190–197

Eliahou H E, Silverberg D S, Reisin E, Roman I, Mashiach S, Serr D M 1978 Propranolol for the treatment of hypertension in pregnancy. British Journal of Obstetrics and Gynaecology 85: 431–436

European Dialysis and Transplant Association 1980 Successful pregnancies in women treated by dialysis and kidney transplantation. British Journal of Obstetrics and Gynaecology 87: 839–645

Feldman G L, Weaver D D, Lovrien E W 1977 The fetal trimethadione syndrome. American Journal of Diseases in Childhood 131: 1389–1392

Fisher D A, Dussault J H, Sack J, Chopra I J 1977 Ontogenesis of hypothalamic-pituitary-thyroid function and metabolism in man, sheep and rat. Recent Progress in Hormone Research 33: 59–116

Gallery E D M, Saunders D M, Hunyor S N, Györy A Z 1979 Randomised comparison of methyldopa and oxprenolol for treatment of hypertension in pregnancy. British Medical Journal i: 1591–1594

Gardiner-Hill H 1929 Pregnancy complicating simple goitre and Grave's disease. Lancet i: 120–124

Goldie L 1974 The role of the psychiatrist in obstetric therapeutics. In: Hawkins D F (editor) Obstetric therapeutics, Baillière-Tindall, London, pp 190–214.

Goodenday L S, Gordan G S 1971 No risk from vitamin D in pregnancy. Annals of Internal Medicine 75: 807–808

Hall J G, Pauli R M, Wilson K M 1980 Maternal and fetal sequelae of anticoagulation during pregnancy. American Journal of Medicine 68: 122–140

Halstead C H, Ghandi G, Tanimura T 1981 Sulfasalazine inhibits absorption of folates in ulcerative colitis. New England Journal of Medicine 305: 1513–1517

Hanson J W, Myrianthopoulos N C, Harvey M A S, Smith D W 1976 Risks to the offspring of women treated with hydantoin anticonvulsants, with emphasis on the fetal hydantoin syndrome. Journal of Pediatrics 89: 662–668

Hartz S C, Heinonen O P, Shapiro S, Siskind V, Slone D 1975 Antenatal exposure to meprobamate and chlordiazepoxide in relation to malformations, mental development and childhood mortality. New England Journal of Medicine 292: 726–728

Hawkins D F, Love W 1978 Counselling on the hazards of pregnancy in operating theatre staff. Anaesthesia 33: 96–97

Heinonen O P, Slone D, Shapiro S 1977 Birth defects and drugs in pregnancy. Publishing Sciences Groups, Littleton, Massachusetts

Hirsh J, Cade J F, O'Sullivan E F 1970 Clinical experience with anticoagulant therapy during pregnancy. British Medical Journal i: 270–273

Holdcroft A, Robinson M J, Gordon H, Whitwam J G 1974 Comparison of two induction doses of methohexitone on infants delivered by caesarean section. British Medical Journal ii: 472–475

Holmberg P C 1979 Central-nervous-system defects in children born to mothers exposed to organic solvents in pregnancy. Lancet ii: 177–178

Jacoby H E, Arnot R N, Glass H I, McClure Browne J C 1972 Estimation of clearance rate of inhaled xenon-133 in the placental region of the pregnant uterus. Journal of Obstetrics and Gynaecology of the British Commonwealth 79: 531–537

Johnson T, Clayton C G 1957 Diffusion of radioactive sodium in normal and preeclamptic pregnancies. British Medical Journal i: 312–314

Joupilla P, Joupilla R, Hollmen A, Koivula A 1982 Lumbar epidural analgesia to improve intervillous blood flow during labour in severe pre-eclampsia. Obstetrics and Gynecology 59: 158–161

Kampmann J P, Johansen K, Hansen J M, Helweg J 1980 Propylthiouracil in human milk. Lancet i: 736–737

Larsen J F, Jacobsen B, Holm H H, Pedersen J F, Mantoni M 1978 Intrauterine injection of vitamin K before the delivery during anticoagulant therapy of the mother. Acta obstetricia et gynaecologica Scandinavica 57: 227–230

Leather H M, Humphreys D M, Baker P, Chadd M A 1968 A controlled trial of hypotensive agents in hypertension in pregnancy. Lancet ii: 488–490

Ledward R S, Hawkins D F 1982 Drug Treatment in Obstetrics. Chapman and Hall, London, pp 177–187

Levy W, Wisniewsky K 1974 Chlorpromazine causing extra-pyramidal dysfunction. New York State Journal of Medicine 74: 684–685

Lewis P J, Bulpitt C J, Zuspan F P 1980 A comparison of current British and American practice in the management of hypertension in pregnancy. Journal of Obstetrics and Gynaecology 1: 78–82

Liley A W 1970 Clinical and laboratory significance of variations in maternal plasma volume in pregnancy. International Journal of Gynaecology and Obstetrics 8: 358–362

McCarroll A M, Hutchinson M, McCauley R, Montgomery A D 1976 Long-term assessment of children exposed *in utero* to carbimazole. Archives of Disease in Childhood 51: 532–536

Man E B, Heineman M, Johnson C E, Leary D C, Peters J P 1951 Precipitable iodine of serum in normal pregnancy and its relation to abortions. Journal of Clinical Investigation 30: 137–150

Menzies D N 1964 Controlled trial of chlorothiazide in early pre-eclampsia. British Medical Journal i: 739–742

Milkovich L, van den Berg B J 1974 Effects of prenatal meprobamate and chlordiazepoxide hydrochloride on human embryonic and fetal development. New England Journal of Medicine 291: 1268–1271

Milner R D G, Chouksey S K 1972 Effects of fetal exposure to diazoxide in man. Archives of Disease in Childhood 47: 537–543

Monks A, Boobis S, Wadsworth J, Richens A 1978 Plasma protein binding interaction between phenytoin and valproic acid *in vitro*. British Journal of Clinical Pharmacology 6: 487–492

Morris N 1953 Hexamethonium compounds in the treatment of pre-eclampsia and essential hypertension in pregnancy. Proceedings of the Royal Society of Medicine 46: 402–406

Nishimura H, Tanimura T 1976a, b, c Clinical aspects of the teratogenicity of drugs. Excerpta Medica, Amsterdam and Oxford; Elsevier, New York, pp 6, 220–224 and 259–262 respectively.

Perucca E, Richens A, Ruprah M 1981 Serum protein binding of phenytoin in pregnant women. British Journal of Clinical Pharmacology 11: 409–411P

Redman C W G, Beilin L J, Bonnar J, Ounsted M K 1976 Fetal outcome in trial of antihypertensive treatment in pregnancy. Lancet ii: 753–756

Reynolds E H 1967 Effects of folic acid on the mental state and fit-frequency of drug-treated epileptic patients. Lancet i: 1086–1088

Robson J M, Poulson E, Sullivan F M 1965 Pharmacological principles of teratogenesis. In: Robson J M, Sullivan F M and Smith R L V (editors) Embryopathic activity of drugs. Churchill, London, pp 21–35

Rodriguez S V, Leiken S L, Hiller M C 1974 Neonatal administration of thiazide drugs. New England Journal of Medicine 270: 881–884

Rudolf J E, Schweitzer R T, Bartus S A 1979 Pregnancy in renal transplant patients. Transplantation 27: 26–29

Schou M, Amdisen A, Steenstrup O R 1973b Lithium and pregnancy—II Hazards to women given lithium during pregnancy and delivery. British Medical Journal ii: 137–138

Schou M, Goldfield M D, Weinstein M R, Villeneuve A 1973a Lithium and pregnancy—I, Report from the Register of Lithium Babies. British Medical Journal ii: 135–136

Smith B E 1974 Teratology in anaesthesia. Clinical Obstetrics and Gynecology 17: 145–163

Smithells R W 1976 Environmental teratogens of man. British Medical Bulletin 32: 27–33

Speidel B D, Meadow S R 1972 Maternal epilepsy and abnormalities of the fetus and newborn. Lancet ii: 839–843

Starreveld-Zimmerman A A E, van der Kolk W J, Elshove J, Meinardi H 1974 Teratogenicity of antiepileptic drugs. Clinical Neurology and Neurosurgery 77: 81–95

Stirrat G M, Lieberman B A 1977 Fetal outcome in pregnancies complicated by severe hypertension treated with propranolol. In: Lewis P J (editor) Therapeutic problems in pregnancy. MTP Press, Lancaster, pp 45–41

Sweet D L, Jr, Kinzie J 1976 Consequences of radiotherapy and antineoplastic therapy for the fetus. Journal of Reproductive Medicine 17: 241–246

de Swiet M 1979 Effect of pregnancy on therapeutic management of coincidental diseases. Prescribers' Journal 19: 59–66

Ullery J C 1954 Thromboembolic disease complicating pregnancy and the puerperium. American Journal of Obstetrics and Gynecology 68 1243–1260

Vessey M P, Nunn J F 1980 Occupational hazards of anaesthesia. British Medical Journal 281: 696–698

Villasanta V 1965 Thromboembolic disease in pregnancy. American Journal of Obstetrics and Gynecology 93: 142–160

Weinstein M R 1976 The international register of lithium babies. Drug Information Journal 2: 94–100

Zucker R, Simon G 1968 Prolonged symptomatic neonatal hypoglycaemia associated with maternal chlorpropamide therapy. Pediatrics 42: 824–825

# Sedatives in pregnancy

In making a decision to give a sedative drug to a pregnant woman, the doctor must balance the anticipated benefits against the potential hazards. In early pregnancy the risks are largely those of possible teratogenesis, while in late pregnancy they are those of the unwanted effects of the drug on the newborn infant.

## USE OF SEDATIVES IN THE FIRST TRIMESTER OF PREGNANCY

### Barbiturates

All barbiturates cross the placenta and attain higher levels in fetal tissues than maternal because of limited fetal elimination of these substances (Ploman and Persson 1957, Melchior et al 1967). There is no evidence that low doses of barbiturates are teratogenic.

Nelson and Forfar (1971) made a retrospective survey of the drug consumption of 450 mothers giving birth to babies with malformations and 1000 control mothers. They found a significant increase in malformations in babies of women who had taken barbiturates in pregnancy, but there was no consistent relationship between the drug, the period of gestation at which it had been taken and the nature of the malformation. The prospective survey of 9000 pregnancies by the Royal College of General Practitioners (1975) also showed a marginal excess of women in the group giving birth to malformed babies had taken barbiturates in early pregnancy. Further analysis again showed no consistent relationship between the drug, the time of administration and the abnormality and the conclusion reached was that there was no suggestion of a cause and effect relationship.

In contrast, with mothers on anticonvulsants of all types there is an overall increase in malformations whatever drug regime is used. The risk is two to four times the background risk and debate centres on what proportion of this risk is related to drugs and what proportion to maternal or constitutional factors. Barbiturates alone appear to be less teratogenic than other anticonvulsants but may potentiate the effects of phenytoin (Starreveld-Zimmerman 1973, Fedrick 1973). There are several reports of defects occurring in infants whose mothers were maintained on barbiturate alone (Speidel and Meadow 1972, Lowe 1973).

A syndrome resembling the fetal hydantoin syndrome has been reported in association with massive phenobarbitone dosage in pregnancy (Siep 1976). The affected infants showed dysmorphic facial features, digital hypoplasia and growth retardation. Dysmorphic facial features have also been reported in infants whose mothers were on barbiturate only (Béthenod and Frédérich 1975).

Folic acid deficiency has been suggested as the mechanism by which both barbiturates and phenytoin may be associated with fetal anticonvulsant syndrome (Siep 1976).

**Benzodiazepines**

*Diazepam* passes rapidly to the fetus and when administered in early pregnancy reaches higher levels in cord plasma than maternal plasma (Shannon et al 1972). Tissue levels in the fetal gastro-intestinal tract, liver and particularly brain remain high. The fetus cannot metabolise diazepam to any appreciable extent (Morselli et al 1973).

There have been three studies relating maternal diazepam ingestion in early pregnancy to the development of oral clefts in babies. Safra and Oakley (1975) interviewed 278 women who had given birth to babies with various malformations. Diazepam ingestion was four times more frequent in mothers of infants with cleft lip (with or without cleft palate) than among mothers of infants with other defects. The mothers' drug consumption was ascertained by interview and not verified in any way; several of the mothers of infants with cleft lips had taken at least one other drug during the first trimester. Saxen and Saxen (1975), using the Finnish Register of congenital malformations and maternal welfare centre records, showed a significant association between benzodiazepine ingestion during the first trimester of pregnancy and oral clefts in infants; 25 of 464 mothers of infants with oral clefts compared with 9 of 456 control mothers had taken benzodiazepine in early pregnancy as indicated on maternity records. Aarskog (1975) sent questionnaires to 130 mothers of infants with oral clefts and reported a 6.1 per cent rate of exposure to diazepam in mothers of babies with cleft lip (with or without cleft palate). The first trimester exposure rate for the general population (determined from antenatal records) was 1.1 per cent.

The interpretation of all three studies must be affected by their retrospective nature. The use of diazepam trebled in the United States over the period of the Safra and Oakley study but no increase in the incidence of oral clefts was shown. If there is an increased risk of oral clefts with first trimester diazepam ingestion it is low—about two to four times the background risk of 0.1 per cent. It must be admitted that if the association was causal, doubling the first trimester exposure rate to diazepam would increase the incidence of cleft lip (with or without cleft palate) only by about 5 per cent, which would not be detected as significant.

*Chlordiazepoxide*. A prospective epidemiological study of 1900 pregnancies (Milkovich and van den Berg 1974) showed a fourfold increase in malformations in babies whose mothers had taken chlordiazepoxide or meprobamate in early pregnancy. However a study comparing 1870 children exposed to chlordiazepoxide in early prenatal life with 48 000 children with no exposure to the drug showed no increase in malformations or mental or motor impairment at later testing (Hartz et al 1975). Another survey of 22 000 pregnancies showed no adverse effect of chlordiazepoxide ingestion in early pregnancy, although there was a slight excess of women bearing children with malformations among those who had taken meprobamate (Crombie et al 1975).

## Phenothiazines

There are several isolated reports of defects, particularly of the limbs, associated with maternal ingestion of phenothiazines in early pregnancy. A prospective study of 50 000 pregnancies showed no difference in birth weight perinatal mortality or intelligence quotient at 4 years in 1309 children exposed to phenothiazines in their first 4 intrauterine months compared with 48 973 not exposed (Slone and Suskind 1977). The suggestion that prenatal exposure to chlorpromazine may cause retinopathy because of the affinity of the drug for melanin containing tissues (Ullberg et al 1970) has not been substantiated.

## Conclusion

While no definite evidence of teratogenesis exists for any drugs discussed, it is possible that their use in early pregnancy may be associated with a small increased risk of malformation over and above the background risk. There is no evidence that the benzodiazepines are less teratogenic than the barbiturates or phenothiazines, which have been used for a considerably longer time.

## USE OF SEDATIVES IN THE SECOND AND THIRD TRIMESTERS OF PREGNANCY

### Barbiturates

Barbiturates of all three types (thiobarbiturates, oxybarbiturates and long acting barbiturates) pass readily to the fetus and attain fetal levels comparable to or higher than maternal levels.

Several studies using Apgar scores as an index have shown the general depressant effect of barbiturates on the newborn when administered to the mother in labour. A restrospective study of 1000 vaginal deliveries divided into three groups—pethidine; pethidine and quinalbarbitone (secobarbital); no medication—showed that babies whose mothers had received both pethidine and quinalbarbitone had significantly more depressed Apgar scores than babies whose mothers had pethidine or no medication (Shnider and Moya 1964). Borgstedt and Rosen (1968) showed no difference in Apgar scores in babies whose mothers had received pethidine or phenobarbitone or nothing. They did show altered electro-encephalographic activity in 30 per cent of the medicated group. Batt (1968) showed that the administration of vinbarbitone (vinbarbital) in labour, with or without phenothiazine, resulted in lower Apgar scores in the newborn and delay in establishing respiration, compared with babies whose mothers had received pethidine alone or with a phenothiazine.

The Apgar score does not assess neonatal behaviour. More complex investigations have shown depressant effects of barbiturate given to the mother in labour on the baby's behaviour. Brazelton (1961) compared the effects of a high dose of barbiturate (> 150 mg) with those of a low dose of barbiturate (< 60 mg) given with either inhalational or local anaesthesia. He found that administration of a high dose of barbiturate 1 to 6 hours before delivery was associated with a less responsive baby with poorer sucking ability and weight gain in both inhalational and local anaesthetic groups. Babies born to mothers given 200 mg of quinalbarbitone between 10 and 180 minutes before delivery had slightly lower Apgar scores but markedly reduced sucking rates, sucking pressures and milk intake. These effects lasted at least 5 days (Kron et al 1966).

Visual attention was reduced in 2 to 4 day old newborn whose mothers had received a variety of drugs, including barbiturate, before delivery. Attentive behaviour was most reduced where the mother had received the highest doses or where the drugs were given within 90 minutes of delivery (Stechler 1964). The long term effects on infant development of the administration of drugs, including barbiturates, to women in labour has been the subject of considerable recent debate (Brackbill 1979). Studies which claim to show such long term effects relate to a variety of drugs in combination with various forms of anaesthesia in a variety of obstetric conditions. It would seem that the mother's personality characteristics in requiring more obstetric medication have more influence on the infant's later development than has the medication itself.

A definite syndrome of barbiturate withdrawal occurs in infants of mothers given barbiturate as a sedative, as an anticonvulsant, or obtained as a drug of addiction (Blumenthal and Lindsay 1977). The clinical features of the syndrome are restlessness, irritability, tremors, hyper-reflexia, shrill cry, sleep disturbance, hyperphagia and vomiting (Desmond et al 1972). Convulsions have been described (Bleyer and Marshall 1972). A less severe form may present with irritability, jitteriness and vomiting. The onset is 3 to 10 days after birth, usually at about 6 days. A subacute phase may last several months with hyperphagia, prolonged crying, hyperacusis and episodic irritability (Desmond et al 1972).

Several authors have described poor later growth in infants of mothers on barbiturates in pregnancy. This appears to be related to feeding difficulties rather than intra-uterine growth retardation, although the latter has been described in babies of mothers on anticonvulsants (Siep 1976, Béthénod and Frédérich 1975).

The role of phenobarbitone as an enzyme inducer has both advantages and disadvantages for the infant. By inducing the activity of the enzyme glucuronyl transferase, phenobarbitone promotes the excretion of bilirubin. This takes 3 to 7 days to occur in the term infant and longer in the preterm infant. The effectiveness of phenobarbitone in reducing bilirubin levels in babies when administered to mothers in late pregnancy has been shown (Thomas 1976), but several studies have shown no benefit to the preterm baby where hyperbilirubinaemia is more likely to have long term consequences (Vaisman and Gartner 1975). Controlled trials have shown no advantage in giving phenobarbitone and phototherapy over phototherapy alone (Valdes et al 1971). The enzyme-inducing effect of phenobarbitone may enhance the hepatic clearance of other drugs administered to the infant and may alter vitamin D metabolism and other steroid hydroxylases at a critical period in development (Lathe 1976). Coagulation defects in babies whose mothers are on long term barbiturate (usually as an anticonvulsant) are probably due to combination with phenytoin.

Myers and Myers (1979) have postulated a protective effect of barbiturate on the hypoxic fetus, by four experimentally demonstrated mechanisms: 1. Depression of brain metabolism and reduction of lactic acid production. 2. Reduction of maternal sympathetic nervous system activity and improvement of uterine blood flow. 3. Reduction of uterine muscle activity and hence reduction of the hypoxic stress of contractions on the fetus. 4. Reduction of stress induced maternal hyperglycaemia and hence reduction of lactic acid production. These theoretical benefits must be weighed against well recognised hazards of such therapy to a stressed fetus. Myers and Myers amassed considerable evidence on the role of anxiety and psychological stress in fetal outcome in animals and man. One can endorse their plea for more care and support for mothers in labour and the reduction of stressful procedures without encouraging the widespread use of barbiturate as an anti-anxiety agent.

**Benzodiazepines**

Diazepam given to the mother rapidly attains higher levels in the fetus than the mother. The drug accumulates in fetal tissues, particularly in the nervous system. Preterm and term babies have a limited capacity to metabolise diazepam, and active drug and metabolites may persist in the baby for at least 1 to 2 weeks after delivery.

Doses of diazepam of 30 mg or more in the 15 hours before delivery can cause respiratory depression, apnoea, hypotonia, poor feeding and impaired thermogenesis (Cree et al 1973). Smaller doses of diazepam may cause hypotonia and feeding difficulties sufficient to warrant investigation of the infant and its observation in the special care nursery with consequent anxiety for the mother and disruption of breast feeding. Nitrazepam and chlordiazepoxide can cause similar effects when small and regular doses are given to the mother in late pregnancy. The regular administration of these benzodiazepines to mother may result in a neonatal withdrawal syndrome of irritability, jitteriness and poor feeding (Rementería and Bhatt 1977).

**Phenothiazines**

Single doses of phenothiazines in late pregnancy or labour have not been shown to cause any ill-effects on the newborn. Regular phenothiazine treatment using high doses may cause extrapyramidal dysfunction in the newborn which may persist for months (Hill et al 1966). The $\alpha$-sympatholytic action of phenothiazines is a theoretical hazard to the newborn in inhibiting noradrenaline mediated thermogenesis but this effect does not seem to have clinical importance.

## CONCLUSION

We are now more aware of the complex nature of neonatal behaviour and the many abilities of the newborn infant. Neonates can discriminate their mother's face and smell, turn to her voice in preference to other sounds and show preference for complex rather than simple visual patterns. Together with this increasing evidence of the sophistication of neonatal behaviour has come an awareness of the importance of the early hours and days after birth in the developing relationship between mother and baby. The behaviour of the normal full term unsedated infant in turning to its mother's voice and regarding her face promotes maternal attachment and caretaking behaviour from mother which in turn reinforces the baby's responses. Klaus et al (1970) have shown the importance of eye to eye contact during this phase—a form of interaction which is impossible with a heavily sedated infant.

Even small amounts of additional early and dose contact between mother and newborn can favourable influence later maternal behaviour and help the establishment of breast feeding (Kennell et al 1974, Sosa et al 1976). Drugs which interfere with this contact may have effects beyond the immediate neonatal period. Careful studies have shown that small amounts of analgesic or local anaesthetic well timed in labour do not have a detrimental effect on behaviour in full term healthy babies (Lieberman et al 1979). There are no similar studies for benzodiazepines, phenothiazines or barbiturates as these drugs are almost always used in combination with analgesic or anaesthetic agents or where there are obstetric complications such as pre-eclampsia. No sedative is entirely free of effects on the newborn and it would seem prudent to avoid repeated doses of any of this group of drugs in late pregnancy unless good indications exist. In particular, giving regular benzodiazepines to antenatal patients as a 'nightcap' should be avoided.

None of these drugs have effects on the newborn severe enough to prevent their careful use in late pregnancy where there is serious maternal disease. Awareness of the potential effects of these sedatives on the newborn baby should prevent their use for trivial indications.

## REFERENCES

Aarskog D 1975 Association between maternal intake of diazepam and oral clefts. Lancet ii: 291

Batt B L 1968 Are large doses of intravenous barbiturates justified for use as premedication in labour? American Journal of Obstetrics and Gynecology 102: 591–596

Béthénod M Frédérich A 1975 Les enfants des antiépileptiques. Pediatrie 30: 227–248

Bleyer W A Marshall R E 1972 Barbiturate withdrawal syndrome in a passively addicted infant. Journal of the American Medical Association 221: 185–186

Blumenthal I, Lindsay S 1977 Neonatal barbiturate withdrawal. Postgraduate Medical Journal 53: 157–158

Borgstedt A D, Rosen M G 1968 Medication during labour correlated with behaviour and EEG of the newborn. American Journal of Diseases of Children 115: 21–24

Brackbill Y 1979 Obstetric medication survey. Science 205: 447–448

Brazelton T B 1961 Psychophysiologic reactions in the neonate. Effect of maternal medication on the neonate and his behavior. Journal of Pediatrics 58: 513–518

Cree J E, Meyer J, Hailey D M 1973 Diazepam in labour. Its metabolism and effect on clinical condition and thermogenesis of the newborn. British Medical Journal iv: 251–255

Crombie D L, Pinsent R J, Fleming D M, Remeau-Rouquette C, Goujard J, Huel G 1975 Fetal effects of tranquillizers in pregnancy. New England Journal of Medicine 293: 198–199

Desmond M M, Schwanecki R P, Wilson G S, Yasunaga S, Burgdorft I 1972 Maternal barbiturate utilization and neonatal withdrawal symptomatology. Pediatrics 80: 190–197

Fedrick J 1973 Epilepsy and pregnancy. A report from the Oxford record linkage study. British Medical Journal ii: 442–448

Hartz S C Heinonen O P, Shapiro S, Siskind V, Slone D 1975 Antenatal exposure to meprobamate and chlordiazepoxide in relation to malformations mental development and childhood mortality. New England Journal of Medicine 292: 726–728

Hill R M, Desmond M M, Kay J L 1966 Extrapyramidal dysfunction in an infant of a schizophrenic mother. Journal of Pediatrics 69: 589–595

Kennell J H, Jerauld R, Wolfe H, Chester D, Kreger N C, McAlpine W, Steffa M, Klaus M H 1974 Maternal behaviour one year after early and extended postpartum contact. Developmental Medicine and Child Neurology 16: 172–179

Klaus M, Kennell J H Plumb N 1970 Human maternal behaviour at the first contact with her young. Pediatrics 46: 187–192

Kron R E, Stein M, Goddard K E 1966 Newborn sucking behaviour affected by obstetric sedation. Pediatrics 37: 1012–1016

Lathe G H 1976 Neonatal bilirubin metabolism in relation to jaundice. Clinics in Endocrinology and Metabolism 5: 107–122

Liebermann B A, Rosenblatt D B, Belsey E, Packer M, Redshaw M, Mills M, Caldwell J, Notarianni L, Smith R L Williams M, Beard R W 1979 The effects of maternally administered pethidine or epidural bupivicaine on the fetus and newborn. British Journal of Obstetrics and Gynaecology 86: 598–606

Lowe C R 1973 Congenital malformations among infants born to epileptic women. Lancet i: 9–10

Melchior J C, Svensmark O, Trolle D 1967 Placental transfer of phenobarbitone in epileptic women and elimination in newborns. Lancet ii: 860–861

Milkovich L, van den Berg B J 1974 Effects of prenatal meprobamate and chlordiazepoxide hydrochloride on human embryonic and foetal development. New England Journal of Medicine 291: 1268–1271

Morselli P L, Principi N, Tognoni G, Reali E, Belvedere G, Standen S M, Sereni F 1973 Diazepam elimination in premature and full term infants and children. Journal of Perinatal Medicine 1: 133–141

Myers R E, Myers S E 1979 Use of sedative analgesic and anaesthetic drugs during labour and delivery. Bane or boon? American Journal of Obstetrics and Gynecology 133: 83–104

Nelson M M, Forfar J O 1971 Association between drugs administered during pregnancy and congenital abnormalities of the foetus. British Medical Journal i: 523–527

Ploman L, Persson B H 1957 On the transfer of barbiturates to the human foetus and their accumulation in some of its vital organs. Journal of Obstetrics and Gynaecology of the British Empire 64: 706–711

Rementería J L, Bhatt K 1977 Withdrawal symptoms in neonates from intrauterine exposure to diazepam. Journal of Pediatrics 90: 123–126

Royal College of General Practitioners 1975 Morbidity and drugs in pregnancy. The influence of illness and drugs on the aetiology of congenital malformations. Journal of the Royal College of General Practitioners 25: 631–645

Safra M J, Oakley G P 1975 Association between cleft lip with or without cleft palate and prenatal exposure to diazepam. Lancet ii: 478–479

Saxen I, Saxen L 1975 Association between maternal intake of diazepam and oral clefts. Lancet ii: 498

Shannon R W, Fraser G P, Aitken R G 1972 Diazepam in pre-eclamptic toxaemia with special reference to its effect on the newborn infant. British Journal of Clinical Practice 26: 271–275

Shnider S M, Moya F 1964 Effects of meperidine on the newborn infant. American Journal of Obstetrics and Gynecology 89: 1009–1015

Siep M 1976 Growth retardation, dysmorphic facies and minor malformations following massive exposure to phenobarbitone in utero. Acta Paediatrica Scandinavica 65: 617–621

Slone D, Suskind V 1977 Antenatal exposure to the phenothiazines in relation to congenital malformations perinatal mortality birth weight and IQ score. American Journal of Obstetrics and Gynecology 128: 486–488

Sosa R, Klaus M, Kennell J H, Urrutia J J 1976 The effect of early mother infant contact on breast feeding infection and growth. In: Breast feeding and the mother. Ciba Foundation Symposium 45. Amsterdam, Elsevier, pp 179–192

Spiedel B D, Meadow S R 1972 Maternal epilepsy and abnormalities of the fetus and newborn. Lancet ii: 839–843

Starreveld-Zimmerman A A E, van der Kolk W T, Elshove J, Meinardi H 1973 Teratogenicity of anti epileptic drugs. Clinical Neurology and Neurosurgery 77: 81

Stechler G 1964 Newborn attention as affected by medication during labour. Science 144: 315

Thomas C R 1976 Routine phenobarbital for prevention of neonatal hyperbilirubinaemia. Obstetrics and Gynecology 47: 304–308

Ullberg S, Lindquist N G, Sjostrand S E 1970 Accumulation of chorioretinotoxic drugs in the foetal eye. Nature 227: 1257–1258

Vaisman S L, Gartner L M 1975 Pharmacologic treatment of neonatal hyperbilirubinemia. Clinics in Perinatology 2: 37–57

Valdes D S, Maurer A M, Shumway C N 1971 Controlled trial of phenobarbital and/or light in reducing neonatal hyperbilirubinemia in a predominantly Negro population. Journal of Pediatrics 79: 1015–1017

*R.S. Ledward*

# Antimicrobial drugs in pregnancy

The general principles of antimicrobial therapeutics apply in pregnancy, but additional factors influence treatment. The physiological adaptations of pregnancy may alter the pharmacokinetics of the drugs, for example, by affecting absorption or metabolism. The other important consideration is the fetus. Whilst in general administration of an antibiotic will benefit the fetus, occasionally the effect may be detrimental.

## PLACENTAL TRANSFER OF ANTIBIOTICS

Nearly all antibiotics cross the placenta by simple diffusion from a high to a low concentration. The rate of transfer is related to the concentration gradient and to the thickness and surface area of the placental membrane, as well as a characteristic diffusion constant for the drug concerned. The quantity of drug transferred per unit time to the fetus is given by Fick's equation as $K.A.(C_m - C_f)/L$, where K is the diffusion constant, A the area of the placental membrane, $C_m$ and $C_f$ the concentrations of free drug in maternal and fetal plasma, respectively, and L the transplacental distance. The diffusion constant is related inversely to the molecular weight of the drug and also to the spatial configuration of its molecules. Molecules with a molecular weight less than 1500 normally pass the placenta by simple diffusion. Highly fat soluble molecules that are uncharged reach the fetus more rapidly than ionised drugs with low fat solubility.

Pharmacokinetic information on the transfer of antibiotics to the fetus is limited. Results obtained in animals which have different placental structures are of questionable applicability. A certain amount of information is available from human pregnancies terminated early, but the results cannot be extrapolated with certainty to late pregnancy. A fairly good source of information is probably cord blood after the mother has been given a parenteral antibiotic in labour.

Nonetheless, some drugs accumulate in organs to levels well above those in plasma, and the possibility exists that selected antibiotics could be used for intra-uterine fetal therapeutics. On the other hand therapeutic levels in amniotic fluid may not be achieved for 4 to 6 hours after administration of an antibiotic to the mother (Duignan et al 1973). The amniotic fluid level is primarily related to renal excretion of the drug by the fetus (Bernard et al 1977)

Nan and Liddiard (1978) give a table of placental transfer of drugs in the first half of human pregnancy showing the relation between maternal blood concentration of a number of antimicrobial agents and the concentration in fetal tissues. A table showing fetal concentrations of antibiotics given to the mother in late pregnancy is given in Ledward and Hawkins (1982).

## PRINCIPLES OF ANTIMICROBIAL TREATMENT IN OBSTETRICS

Attitudes to antimicrobial treatment in pregnancy are affected by the nature of the patient population, by the tendency of severe infections in pregnancy to develop rapidly, by the need to protect the fetus and by concern for preservation of the patient's future fertility.

### Selection of drugs

In general, pregnant women are drawn from a healthy segment of the population who have not had repeated courses of antibiotics and who do not harbour resistant bacteria. Well-known antibiotics which have been used for years are usually effective and more recent drugs can be reserved for infections that do not respond. There is little indication to use the latest trivial molecular modification whose side effects in pregnancy are ill-documented.

### Initiation of treatment

Bacteriological investigations must be requested immediately infection is diagnosed. With a high pyrexia, blood cultures should be included; genital tract swabs need anaerobic as well as aerobic culture. Treatment with moderately large doses of antimicrobial drugs is then started, without waiting for the bacteriological results. The drugs are selected either with an educated guess at the responsible organism, or with severe infection, to cover a wide spectrum of organisms. If broad spectrum treatment is indicated, there are three main groups of organisms to be considered—Gram positive bacteria, Gram negative bacteria and anaerobes. With continued treatment, disturbance of endogenous flora will occur, and B vitamins should be administered and oral and vaginal antifungal treatment given. With prolonged intravenous regimens, local antifungal preparations should be used round intravenous infusion sites and intravenous catheters cultured when they are removed.

The practice of completely revising an antimicrobial regimen directly bacteriological sensitivities become available is highly undesirable. The clinical response of the patient is a better indicator of the sensitivity of pathogens than any laboratory bacteriological test. To change the antibiotic to which the patient is responding delays treatment by up to 24 hours and is conducive to bacterial resistance. Change in the regimen, preferably by addition of another drug, is indicated by failure of clinical response within 24 to 48 hours. The selection of the additional agent is then guided by the laboratory sensitivities of the organisms isolated.

It is desirable when giving combinations of antibotics to give a bactericidal agent with a bacteriostatic drug. This is not always easy to apply in practice, as many bactericidal drugs are bacteriostatic in lower concentrations or when used against relatively resistant organisms. When the presence of a haemolytic streptococcus, a pneumococcus or *Clostridium welchii* is suspected, benzylpenicillin should be included in the combination. Combinations frequently employed in pregnancy incorporate 1. benzylpenicillin, amoxycillin, flucloxacillin or a cephalosporin such as cefoxitin to deal with Gram positive bacteria 2. sulphadimidine, co-trimoxazole or gentamicin for Gram negative bacteria, and 3. metronidazole if the presence of an anaerobe is suspected. Clindamycin is usually reserved for infections due to resistant organisms or severe infections with anaerobes.

**Route of administration**

Oral administration is reasonable with ordinary infections in relatively well patients. The gastric irritability of pregnant women may cause difficulties; administration of capsules or tablets with a draught of fluid may help. If vomiting occurs then parenteral administration is necessary. In labour, when absorption must be assumed to be much reduced, or in severe infections, the parenteral route is also indicated. There is no evidence that intermittent bolus injections of an antimicrobial drug convey any advantage and the objective is to attain a sustained blood level of the drug.

Infection in a hollow viscus is treated more effectively by systemic administration than by an agent in the lumen. Exceptions have to be made where systemic toxicity limits the effective dose. An example is the use of local fungicides in vaginal thrush.

The comfort of patients is important in selecting routes of administration. Intramuscular benzylpenicillin 6 hourly is painful; procaine penicillin 12 hourly causes much less discomfort and gives better blood levels. To maintain an intravenous drip just to permit 12 hourly intravenous injection of a drug which could be run in through a small vein in 30 minutes is unreasonable.

## CONTRAINDICATIONS TO ANTIMICROBIAL DRUGS IN PREGNANCY

Hypersensitivity implies either allergic sensitivity, usually generated by a previous exposure, or an idiosyncratically low threshold for a toxic effect. Allergic reactions usually take the form of skin reactions, gastro-intestinal intolerance, bronchospasm or anaphylaxis, but may occur as hepatic, neurological, haematological, renal or psychiatric reactions, or even as 'serum sickness' type systemic reactions. Idiosyncratic hypersensitivity may affect almost any organ system—a most unpleasant example is the, fortunately relatively rare, marrow aplasia, leucopenia and thrombocytopenia which can be caused by chloramphenicol. Only a history of intolerance to an antimicrobial drug or closely related agents can indicate in advance that the drug may be contraindicated.

Direct toxic effects of antimicrobial drugs manifest when some factor leads to abnormally high concentrations of the drug. For example, gastro-intestinal disturbances can result from local irritation due to oral preparations of chloramphenicol, lincomycin or tetracycline. Streptomycin instilled intraperitoneally can cause neuromuscular block of respiratory muscles. Parenteral preparations can cause pain or thrombophlebitis locally if dilution or systemic distribution are inadequate. Neurotoxicity and otoxicity can result from unduly high concentrations of aminoglycosides; nephrotoxicity can occur with aminoglycosides, amphotericin, colistin and even, occasionally, with cephalosporins. In all these instances, defective renal excretion is the usual predisposing factor. The older sulphonamides, given with inadequate fluids, could cause crystalluria and consequent renal damage. Excessive dose can be a cause of toxicity—large amounts of tetracycline, more than 2 g/day, have caused hepatic necrosis and death in pregnant woman (Finn and Horwitz 1965). Prevention of direct toxic effects of antimicrobial drugs contraindicates any use that may cause local or systemic overdose.

Teratogenic effects are really direct toxic actions on the developing fetus of agents which pass the placenta freely. The common example is that of tetracyclines. These cause discolouration and defective formation of the deciduous teeth of the developing fetus

(Kline et al 1964). Aminoglycosides can be ototoxic to the fetus. In addition, sulphonamides and novobiocin can pass through to the fetus and, if used shortly before delivery, predispose to neonatal jaundice. Any antimicrobial agent which can interfere with folic acid absorption and metabolism must be considered a theoretical hazard to the fetus unless given with folic acid supplements.

Biological alterations in the host (Yusuf 1976) may result from antibiotic treatment. In particular, treatment with broad spectrum agents may eradicate normal flora and predispose to fungal infections and superinfection with resistant organisms.

There are thus a number of relative contraindications to the use of any antimicrobial drugs, but the clinical need for treating infections is of much greater importance. The best answers to this conflict are careful selection of the most appropriate drugs and careful monitoring of their use.

## AGENTS IN COMMON USE IN PREGNANCY

*Penicillins*. These have been used in pregnancy extensively and seen to be harmless to the fetus. If the mother has some history of a hypersensitivity reaction, a cephalosporin may be used instead, but there is some degree of cross-reaction. Accordingly if there is a clear history of a serious reaction to penicillin, cephalosporins also should be avoided. Penicillin is the best agent in haemolytic streptococcal, pneumococcal, clostridial, gonorrhoeal and syphilitic infections. Amoxycillin is used to treat pyelonephritis in pregnancy. Like ampicillin, it may reduce urinary oestrogen excretion (Tikkanen et al 1973). A concurrent fall in urinary oestriol may not therefore indicate placental insufficiency.

*Cephalosporins*. These have been widely used in pregnancy without apparent harm. They readily pass the placenta and give fetal blood and amniotic fluid levels sufficient to inhibit Gram positive organisms and most strains of Gram negative pathogens commonly encountered in intra-uterine infections (Hirsch 1971, Stewart et al 1973). Cephalexin is a most effective oral agent for urinary infections. If high levels are needed in the fetus in intra-uterine infections parenteral use of β-lactamase resistant cephalosporins such as cefuroxime or cefoxitin is preferable.

*Erythromycin*. This drug may be used for patients who are allergic to penicillin, but relatively low levels are achieved in the fetal circulation when therapeutic doses are given to the mother. This limits the use of erythromycin for fetal infections such as syphilis (Philipson et al 1973). The estolate of erythromycin should be avoided as if administered for more than 10 to 14 days it can give rise to cholestatic jaundice.

*Aminoglycosides*. Gentamicin, kanamycin, neomycin, streptomycin, tobramycin and amikacin are all known to convey a small risk of fetal as well as maternal ototoxicity. If they are used in pregnancy, plasma levels should be monitored. They may be necessary to treat severe genital tract infections in general and septic abortion in particular.

*Tetracyclines*. These should not be prescribed in pregnancy. Alternative antibiotics are always available. Specifically, after 16 weeks maturity they cause discolouration and enamel hypoplasia in the fetal deciduous teeth (Ravid and Toaff 1972). Retarded growth of the fetal fibula can also occur. Rarely tetracyclines can cause fatty necrosis of the liver, pancreatitis and renal damage (Weinstein and Dalton 1968).

*Clindamycin* may be needed in an anaerobic soft tissue infection. Rarely, pseudomembranous colitis due to superinfection with *Clostridium difficile* occurs, requiring treatment with vancomycin.

*Chloramphenicol* is also used in anaerobic infections, but its rare side effect of aplastic anaemia can be lethal, and in general the use of metronidazole is preferred.

*Novobiocin* is rarely used (Gilman et al 1979). Given in late pregnancy it can cause neonatal jaundice (Sutherland and Keller 1961) or thrombocytopenia (Day et al 1958). The jaundice is probably mainly due to interference with bilirubin conjugation (Done 1964).

*Sulphonamides*. Rapid placental transfer occurs and the drugs should not be used in suspected premature labour or in late pregnancy when labour is imminent. A high concentration in the fetus may displace bilirubin from binding sites on the plasma proteins, predisposing to neonatal jaundice with a high free plasma bilirubin, though kernicterus has not been reported. The risk of jaundice is greater in preterm babies with incompletely developed liver and kidney function (Tuchmann-Duplessis 1975). Sulphonamides must also be avoided in patients with glucose-6-phosphate dehydrogenase deficiency; given in late pregnancy they may then cause methaemoglobinaemia in the newborn.

Soluble sulphonamides have been of great use in the treatment of urinary tract infections in pregnancy, though many strains of *E. coli* are now resistant.

Co-trimoxazole (sulphamethoxazole and trimethoprim) has been found experimentally to interfere with folic acid absorption and metabolism. Though the combination has been used widely in human pregnancy without apparent harm, it is wise to give folic acid supplements (5 to 10 mg daily) in addition. Co-trimoxazole is best avoided in pregnancy when the patient's folic acid status may be impaired by a malabsorption syndrome or by anticonvulsant drugs.

*Metronidazole.* This drug has repeatedly been accused of teratogenicity without any valid evidence (for example, see Moellering 1979). In fact there is good evidence that the drug is not teratogenic in humans (see Morgan 1978) and it is widely used to treat parasite infections such as trichomoniasis and also amoebiasis, and severe bacterial anaerobic infections.

Nonetheless, as a matter of general principle, treatment of asymptomatic trichomoniasis or giardiasis is best deferred until the second trimester, and 10 day courses employed rather than single large dose regimens.

*Nitrofurantoin* given when labour is imminent can pass to the fetus and predispose to neonatal haemolysis (Cohlan 1964).

*Quinine and Chloroquine.* High doses of quinine have been thought to cause abortion by a direct action on the myometrium or by a toxic action on the fetus. Ill-effects on the fetus are rare with normal doses. Chloroquine had been reported to be associated with fetal retinal damage but cases are very rare. With either drug, effective treatment of malaria is much more important for the protection of the fetus than any teratogenic hazard.

## MANAGEMENT OF INFECTIONS

### Urinary tract infections

Asymptomatic bacteriuria in pregnancy has been shown to be associated with low birth weight babies (Grüneberg et al 1969), though this may in part be a reflection of the association between low socioeconomic status and bacteriuria (Turck et al 1962). If culture of a mid-stream specimen of urine in early pregnancy yields a pathogen but less than $10^5$ organisms/ml, then a liberal fluid intake should be advised and the culture repeated at intervals. More than $10^5$ organisms/ml calls for a 10 day course of a short acting sulphonamide or of amoxycillin, in the first instance. If bacteriuria persists, treatment is indicated by laboratory sensitivities.

Symptomatic urinary tract infections require active treatment. Whilst awaiting bacteriological results the first choice of agent lies between sulphonamide, amoxycillin and nitrofurantoin. When *in vitro* sensitivities become available, the antimicrobial agent should not be changed if there is clinical response. If the infection fails to respond then another antibiotic, selected according to sensitivities, should be added to the regimen.

## Premature rupture of the membranes

The incidence is quoted as 7 to 12 per cent (Gunn et al 1970), but the term is ill-defined (British Medical Journal 1979), and is best related to the maturity of the pregnancy.

After 34 weeks maturity, there is little doubt that the best management of premature rupture of the membranes is to induce labour, using oxytocin if necessary. Delivery of the baby is the best way of preventing neonatal infection.

With preterm rupture of the membranes before 34 weeks, the onset of premature labour may follow. Vaginal interference should be restricted to a minimum, with a speculum examination to obtain a high vaginal swab for culture, and, if necessary, a single vaginal examination to ascertain cervical dilatation and effacement. Routine prophylactic antibiotics are not usually advised. If they are used without clinical or bacteriological evidence of infection, antibiotic resistance and superimposed candidiasis can occur (Habel et al 1972).

If an infection is suspected, oral amoxycillin or a cephalosporin together with metronidazole are useful. In labour the cephalosporin and metronidazole can be given parenterally. For florid infections benzylpenicillin or cefoxitin can be used with gentamicin.

## Surgical procedures

There is no indication to use routine antimicrobial prophylaxis for such procedures as cervical cerclage, amniocentesis or internal fetal monitoring, and they are best reserved for cases where infection is suspected or would constitute an unusual hazard. Recently the employment of metronidazole prophylaxis for caesarean section has been advocated (Study Group 1978), and this might become accepted practice in centres where anaerobic infections are common.

## Amniotic infection

Amniotic fluid contains immunoglobulin G (Derrington and Soothill 1961), lysozyme (Galask and Snyder 1970) and β-lysin (Ford et al 1981). It supports bacterial growth poorly (Miller et al 1976), perhaps because of a zinc-peptide antibacterial system (Schlievert et al 1976). In the presence of meconium, Gram negative organisms grow freely (Galask and Snyder 1968).

Chorio-amnionitis associated with intra-uterine fetal pneumonia was described by Blanc (1959). The condition is not necessarily related to prematurely ruptured membranes. The incidence of amnionitis has been found to be related to low socio-economic status and to race (Naeye and Blanc 1970). Congenital pneumonia was found in 23 per cent of autopsies on stillborn and newborn babies by Naeye et al (1971). The pneumonia has been considered as secondary to aspiration of amniotic fluid containing leucocytes (Davies 1965, Olding 1966), and thought not to be susceptible to antibiotic treatment (Lebherz et al 1963). If the fetus dies, levels of antibiotics in antibiotic fluid after maternal administration are much reduced (Bray et al 1966), in the absence of fetal renal excretion. If the membranes rupture, replacement of amniotic fluid would be expected to reduce antimicrobial activity, endogenous or therapeutic, by dilution, and predispose to ascending infection.

## Septic abortion

Sepsis is more likely to occur in second trimester abortions, whether spontaneous or induced. The presence of an intra-uterine contraceptive device may predispose to bacteraemia and septicaemic shock (Santamarina and Smith 1970). Treatment should be commenced with parenteral antibiotics to cover both Gram positive and negative organisms, before any surgical interference to evacuate retained products of conception. Appropriate choices of drugs include intravenous ampicillin or a cephalosporin, and kanamycin or gentamicin, together with metronidazole or clindamycin to deal with anaerobic infection. Estimates of the blood levels of the aminoglycoside chosen are helpful. Organisms likely to be involved are aerobic and anaerobic streptococci, staphylococci, enterococci, *E. coli*, *Bacteroides* and *Proteus*.

## Prophylactic use of antibiotics

*Maternal heart disease.* To prevent subacute bacterial endocarditis, antibiotics should be given to women with valvular lesions or septal defects admitted in labour or before surgical induction of labour or caesarean section. Benzylpenicillin, amoxycillin or a cephalosporin such as cephazolin (Hannay et al 1975), may be used but a broad spectrum cover with gentamicin as well is probably better. The antibiotic should be started 6 to 12 hours before surgical interference to allow therapeutic levels to be obtained in the fetus and amniotic fluid as well as the maternal tissues.

Other indications which have been suggested for prophylactic use of antimicrobial agents include repeated vaginal examinations in labour, rupture of the membranes for more than 24 hours, diabetics in labour and intrapartum maternal pyrexia of unknown cause.

## Maternal infections

*Pneumonia*. Penicillin is indicated for pneumococcal disease; flucloxacillin and gentamicin are best for pneumonia complicating influenza.

*Tuberculosis*. All patients with tuberculosis under treatment in pregnancy have a slightly increased risk of fetal abnormality. Studies with rifampicin and ethambutol, the drugs currently favoured, suggest that the risk is no greater with these drugs, even if used in the first trimester, than with other regimens (Jentgens 1973).

Streptomycin used in high doses conveys some risk of ototoxicity of the fetus, and blood levels should be monitored. There may be some delays in passage of the drug through the placenta, resulting in a concentration in fetal blood less than 50 per cent of that in maternal blood (Sakula 1954). This author refers to reports suggesting that streptomycin is innocuous to the fetus, but Leroux (1950) described a single case of a mother receiving 1 g/day of streptomycin for the last month of pregnancy with a baby having auditory impairment at 2½ months of age. In general there is little risk to hearing in the child and any defect of vestibular function is usually compensated, but a significant number of children have some high frequency loss, above the usual auditory range.

Although there are theoretical grounds for thinking that isoniazid might interfere with pyridoxine metabolism, no congenital abnormalities were reported in 93 babies born to women treated with the drug in pregnancy (Lowe 1964, Marcus 1967). Nonetheless it is wise to give pyridoxine supplements (50 mg daily).

*Gonorrhoea; syphilis*. These are best treated by specialised clinics which can follow up contacts. For gonorrhoea, 1 g of probenecid is given orally, followed after 30 minutes with 4.8 Mu procaine penicillin, divided into two doses injected at different intramuscular sites. For syphilis 0.6 to 0.9 Mu of procaine penicillin is given intramuscularly daily for 10 days. A cephalosporin or erythromycin is used in penicillin sensitive patients.

*Listeriosis*. The presence of *L. monocytogenes* in the faeces of a pregnant patient does not necessarily indicate treatment, since the ratio of clinical infection to carriage is very low (Larsson et al 1979). Infections should be treated with amoxycillin, preferably with gentamicin, as the organism can be lethal in the newborn.

*Group B β-haemolytic streptococci* in the vagina only present a hazard to the baby between the time the membranes are ruptured and delivery. In units where there have been neonatal infections with this organism, which may be lethal, it is wise to culture high vaginal swabs from patients where surgical induction of labour is intended. The best protection against colonisation of the baby is then parenteral benzyl penicillin given to the mother throughout labour.

*Fungal infections*

*Candida albicans* is probably a normal commensal in the vagina and causes infections in 10 per cent of pregnant women (Hurley et al 1974). Infection is more likely after the use of broad spectrum antibiotics or steroid treatment and in diabetics. The best treatment is still with nystatin pessaries; the drug may be given orally as well in resistant cases where *Candida* can be cultured from the faeces. Other drugs used include candicidin, clotrimazole, econazole and miconazole.

Systemic infection with *Coccidioides immitis* is extremely rare but it can cause serious maternal illness, abortion, preterm delivery or stillbirth. Treatment is with intravenous amphotericin (Stevenson 1973).

*Protozoal infections*

*Trichomoniasis* in pregnancy is treated with oral metronidazole. Concurrent abstinence from alcohol is advised.

*Malaria* prevention may be important in pregnancy. For most of Africa, the Middle East, Pakistan and India, pyrimethamine 50 mg once a week is given with folic acid 5 mg daily. In Eastern India, Bangladesh, South-east Asia and Central and South America, the best prophylaxis in pregnancy is pyrimethamine 12.5 mg with dapsone 100 mg, twice weekly, and folic acid supplements. Treatment of active malaria in pregnancy is with chloroquine, or in chloroquine-resistant areas, with quinine. The need to protect both mother and fetus far outweighs any very small risk of the fetus being affected by these drugs.

*Amoebiasis* in pregnancy is treated with metronidazole.

*Toxoplasmosis.* In Great Britain, 1 woman in 300 may become infected during pregnancy (Ruoss and Bourne 1972); the laboratory work that would be involved in routine antenatal screening would be considerable. If the only evidence of infection is a positive serum titre, treatment may be with spiramycin, which does not pass the placenta. If the titre rises or there are clinical manifestations, pyrimethamine, dapsone and co-trimoxazole are used with folic acid supplements.

## CONCLUSION

In humans, the antibiotics used routinely may be considered fairly safe for the fetus. Adverse reports relate mainly to anecdotal cases or to animal studies. Antibiotic therapy should not be withheld during pregnancy if it is indicated. Most pharmaceutical manufacturers now protect themselves with their drug inserts stating 'safety for use during pregnancy has not been established'. The doctor has to balance the risk of exposing a fetus to an antibiotic with that of not using the drug to treat an infection in a pregnant patient. If he avoids tetracycline and uses well-known antibiotics instead of the latest molecular modification he is unlikely to place the fetus at risk.

Considerations about infections in pregnancy such as aetiology, diagnosis, prevention and control of viral and other infections, neonatal problems and economic consequences have been extensively discussed by Coid (1977).

More research to determine the concentration in fetal tissues of antimicrobial drugs given to the mother is long overdue. Such knowledge might increase the possibility of intra-uterine fetal therapeutics.

## REFERENCES


Bernard B, Garcia-Cázares S J, Ballard C A, Thrupp L D, Mathies A W, Wehrle P F 1977 Tobramycin: maternal-fetal pharmacology. Antimicrobial Agents and Chemotherapy 11: 688–694

Blanc W A 1959 Amniotic infection syndrome. Clinical Obstetrics and Gynecology 2: 705–734

Bray R E, Boe R W, Johnson W L 1966 Transfer of ampicillin into fetus and amniotic fluid from maternal plasma in late pregnancy. American Journal of Obstetrics and Gynecology 96: 938–942

British Medical Journal 1979. Premature rupture of the membranes. British Medical Journal i: 1165–1166

Cohlan S Q 1964 Foetal and neonatal hazards from drugs administered during pregnancy. New York Journal of Medicine 64: 493–499

Coid C R (editor) 1977 Infections and pregnancy. Academic Press, London, pp. 1, 343, 437, 551

Davies P A 1965 Congenital pneumonia. Clinics in Pediatrics 4: 523–528

Day H J, Conrad F G, Moore J E 1958 Immunothrombocytopenia induced by novobiocin. American Journal of the Medical Sciences 236: 475–482

Derrington M M and Soothill J F 1961 Journal of Obstetrics and Gynaecology of the British Commonwealth 68: 755–761

Done A K 1964 Developmental pharmacology. Clinical Pharmacology and Therapeutics 5: 432–479

Duignan N M, Andrews J, Williams J D 1973 Pharmacological studies with lincomycin in late pregnancy. British Medical Journal iii: 75–78

Finn W F, Horwitz S T 1965 Maternal death due to fatty metamorphosis of liver following tetracycline therapy. New York Journal of Medicine 65: 662–627

Ford L C, Kash W, Heins Y, De Lange R J, Wright J D, Alexander G, Lebherz T B 1981 Identification of β-lysin as a zinc-dependent antibacterial protein in amniotic fluid. Journal of Obstetrics and Gynaecology 2: 79–84.

Galask R P, Snyder I S 1968 Bacterial inhibition by amniotic fluid. American Journal of Obstetrics and Gynecology 102: 949–955

Galask R P, Snyder I S 1970 Antimicrobial factors in amniotic fluid. American Journal of Obstetrics and Gynecology 106: 59–65

Gilman A G, Goodman L S, Gilman D (editors) 1979 The pharmacological basis of therapeutics, 6th edition, Chapter 54, p. 1230

Gunn G C, Mishell D R, Morton D G 1970 Premature rupture of the fetal membranes. American Journal of Obstetrics and Gynecology 106: 469–483

Grüneberg R N, Leigh D A, Brumfitt W 1969 Relationship of bacteriuria in pregnancy to acute pyelonephritis, prematurity and fetal mortality. Lancet ii: 1–3

Habel A H, Sandor G S, Conn N K, McCrae W M 1972 Premature rupture of membranes and effects of prophylactic antibiotic. Archives of Disease in Childhood 47: 401–404

Hannay W T, Sharp F, Parman M G, McAllister T A 1975 Cephazolin in obstetrics. Scottish Medical Journal 20: 175–177

Hirsch H A 1971 The use of cephalosporin antibiotics in pregnant women. Postgraduate Medical Journal 47 (Supplement): 90–93

Hurley R, Stanley V C, Leas B G S, De Louvois J 1974 In: Skinner F A, Carr J G (editors) The normal microbial flora of man. Academic Press, London and New York, p. 155–185

Jentgens H 1973 Antituberkulose Chemotherapie und Schwangerschaftsabruch. Praxis der Pneumologie 27: 479–488

Kline A H, Blattner R J, Lunin M 1964 Transplacental effect of tetracyclines on teeth. Journal of the American Medical Association 188: 178–180

Larsson S, Cronberg S, Winblad S 1979 Listeriosis during pregnancy and neonatal period in Sweden 1958–1974. Acta paediatrica Scandinavica 68: 486–493

Lebherz T B, Hellman L P, Madding R, Anctil A, Arje S L 1963 Double-blind study of premature rupture of the membranes. American Journal of Obstetrics and Gynecology 87: 218–225

Ledward R S, Hawkins D F 1982 Drug treatment in obstetrics. A handbook of prescribing. Chapman and Hall, London, pp 132–134

Leroux M L 1950 Existe-t-il une surdité congénitale acquise due à la strepto-mycine ? Annales d'oto-laryngologie 67: 194–196

Lowe C R 1964 Congenital defects among children born to women under supervision or treatment for pulmonary tuberculosis. British Journal of Preventive and Social Medicine 18: 14–16

Marcus J C 1967 Non teratogenicity of antituberculous drugs. South African Medical Journal 41: 758–759

Miller J, Michel J, Bercovici B, Argaman M, Sacks T 1976 Studies on the antimicrobial activity of amniotic fluid. American Journal of Obstetrics and Gynecology 125: 212–214

Moellering R C 1979 Special consideration of the use of antimicrobial agents during pregnancy, post partum and in the newborn. Clinical Obstetrics and Gynecology 22: 373–378

Morgan I 1978 Metronidazole treatment in pregnancy. International Journal of Gynaecology and Obstetrics 15: 501–502

Naeye R L, Blanc W A 1970 Relation of poverty and race to antenatal infection. New England Journal of Medicine 283: 555–56

Naeye R L, Dellinger W S, Blanc W A 1971 Fetal and maternal features of antenatal bacterial infections. Journal of Pediatrics 79: 733–739

Nan H, Liddiard C 1978 Part IV. In: Neubert D, Merker H J, Nail H, Langman

J (editors) Role of pharmacokinetics in prenatal and perinatal toxicology. Georg Thieme, Stuttgart
Olding L 1966 Bacterial infection in cases of perinatal death. Acta paediatrica Scandinavica 56: Supplement 171, 7–104
Philipson A, Sabath L D, Charles D 1973 Transplacental passage of erythromycin and clindamycin. New England Journal of Medicine 288: 1219–1221
Ravid R, Toaff R 1972 On the possible teratogenicity of antibiotic drugs administered during pregnancy. Advances in Experimental Medicine and Biology 27: 505–509
Ruoss C F, Bourne G L 1972 Toxoplasmosis in pregnancy. Journal of Obstetrics and Gynaecology of the British Commonwealth 79: 1115–1118
Sabath I D 1973 Antibiotics in obstetric practice. In: Charles D, Finland M (editors) Obstetric and perinatal infections, Lea and Febiger, Philadelphia, p. 4
Sakula A 1954 Streptomycin and the foetus. British Journal of Tuberculosis and Diseases of the Chest 48: 69–72.
Santamarina B A G, Smith S A 1970 Septic abortion and septic shock. Clinical Obstetrics and Gynecology 13: 291–304
Schlievert P, Johnson W, Galask R P 1976 Bacterial growth inhibition by amniotic fluid. American Journal of Obstetrics and Gynecology 125: 899–905
Stevenson R E 1973 The foetus and newly born infant. Mosby, St Louis, p. 268
Stewart K S, Shafi M, Andrews J and Williams J D 1973 Distribution of parenteral ampicillin and cephalosporins in late pregnancy. Journal of Obstetrics and Gynaecology of the British Commonwealth 80: 902–908
Study Group 1978 An evaluation of metronidazole in the prophylaxis of anaerobic infections in obstetrical patients. Journal of Antimicrobial Chemotherapy 4 (Supplement C): 55–62
Sutherland J M, Keller W H 1961 Novobiocin and neonatal hyperbilirubinemia. An investigation of the relationship in an epidemic of neonatal hyperbilirubinemia. American Journal of Diseases of Children 101: 447–453
Tikkanen M J, Pulkkinen M O, Adlercreutz H 1973 Effect of ampicillin treatment on the urinary excretion of estriol conjugates in pregnancy. Journal of Steroid Biochemistry 4: 439–440
Tuchman-Duplessis H 1975 Drug effects on the foetus. In: Monographs on drugs 2. Adis Press, New York, chapter 13, Antimicrobial drugs, p 128
Turck M, Goffe B S, Petersdorf R G 1962 Bacteriuria of pregnancy. New England Journal of Medicine 226: 857–860
Weinstein L, Dalton A C 1968 Host determinants of response to antimicrobial agents. New England Journal of Medicine 279: 467–473, 524–531 and 580–587
Yusuf S M 1976 Adverse effects of antimicrobial drugs. Journal of the Pakistan Medical Association 26: 226–229

*R. K. Sidhu*

# Corticosteroids in pregnancy

The absolute indications for the use of corticosteroids in pregnancy are Addison's disease and hypopituitarism. These require strict replacement with doses equivalent to 25 mg per day of cortisone and small doses of a mineralocorticoid such as fludrocortisone to maintain electrolyte balance.

The largest group of patients requiring steroids during pregnancy are those needing treatment for asthma, collagen disease or immunosuppression. Steroid therapy needs close monitoring during pregnancy and it may be necessary to increase the dose in the presence of exacerbation of the disease process for which steroids are being given.

Another group of patients where steroids are used during pregnancy are those who have been given large doses of corticosteroids in the past and in whom there is suspicion of a minor degree of adrenal insufficiency. Many authors have shown evidence of suppression of the hypothalamic-pituitary-adrenal cortex system following administration of steroids. Complete recovery of adrenal function following long term administration of glucocorticoids takes 9 to 12 months in most patients (Graber et al 1965, Livanou et al 1967) but depressed adrenal function can sometimes be demonstrated even years later.

### *Obstetric use of steroids*

Response to steroids in cases of hyperemesis gravidarum who fail to respond to the usual measures may be due to a state of relative adrenal insufficiency which improves as placental steroid production increases. In a series of 29 patients with hyperemesis treated with doses of cortisone varying from 25 to 75 mg/day 23 had a complete remission of symptoms within 36 hours with no recurrence. The total duration of treatment varied from 5 to 64 days, averaging about 3 weeks (Wells 1953).

Corticosteroids have occasionally been used successfully in the very rare case of recurrent missed abortion, occurring repeatedly between 10 and 20 weeks when all the known causes of abortion have been excluded and the hypothesis of an immunological basis for rejection of the conceptus may be entertained (Hawkins, personal communication).

Corticosteroids have been widely used in premature labour. In 1972 Liggins and Howie first demonstrated reduced incidence of respiratory distress syndrome in premature babies after administration of glucocorticoids to the mother. Further prospective controlled trials have confirmed this result (Howie and Liggins 1977, Taeusch et al 1979, Crowley 1981). The efficacy of steroids has been questioned and potential hazards to the fetus and mother suggested (Sachs 1981).

## Drugs available

Relative potency of corticosteroids is usually judged on the basis of their anti-inflammatory and salt retaining potency (Table 10.1). Most of the synthetic glucocorticoids are relatively free of sodium retaining activity though large doses of prednisone or prednisolone may cause such effects. Hydrocortisone has both anti-inflammatory and sodium retaining activities. The commonest glucocorticoids used in pregnancy are prednisolone, betamethasone and dexamethasone. Hydrocortisone is used in an acute situation because of its rapid action.

**Table 10.1** Relative potencies of corticosteroids used in treatment (Sidhu and Hawkins 1981).

| Compound | Relative anti-inflammatory potency | Relative sodium-retaining potency |
|---|---|---|
| Dexamethasone | 25.0 | 0 |
| Betamethasone | 25.0 | 0 |
| Paramethasone | 10.0 | 0 |
| Fludrocortisone | 10.0 | 125.0 |
| Triamcinolone | 5.0 | 0 |
| Methylprednisolone | 5.0 | 0.5 |
| Prednisolone | 4.0 | 0.8 |
| Hydrocortisone | 1.0 | 1.0 |
| Cortisone | 0.8 | 0.8 |

*Prednisolone* is widely used to treat bronchial asthma and collagen disorders. In combination with azathioprine it is used for immunosuppression in patients with renal transplants. Prednisone has the same therapeutic effects as prednisolone.

*Betamethasone* is a potent glucocorticoid and has been used for prevention of respiratory distress syndrome in premature infants (Liggins and Howie 1972). Betamethasone, 0.6 to 0.7 mg, is equivalent in anti-inflammatory activity to 5 mg of prednisone.

*Dexamethasone* is similar in its glucocorticoid potency to betamethasone and is also used in premature labour for prevention of respiratory distress syndrome.

*Hydrocortisone* is used parenterally for conditions such as status asthmaticus and Addisonian crisis, and to prevent or treat circulatory collapse in patients with suppressed adrenal cortex function subjected to stresses such as that of labour.

*Deoxycortone (DOCA) and fludrocortisone* are mineralocorticoids used in replacement therapy for patients with Addison's disease or after adrenalectomy or hypophysectomy. Regular plasma electrolyte estimation should be carried out to monitor the dose during pregnancy.

There is little experience of the use of corticotrophin (ACTH) or the synthetic polypeptide tetracosactrin in pregnancy.

## Management in pregnancy

### *Medical disorders*

Pregnancy outcome in patients with Addison's disease on replacement steroid therapy is usually normal. Some patients with bronchial asthma are taking steroids when they start a pregnancy, and most studies have shown a normal pregnancy outcome in these patients. Beclomethasone inhalation is effective in controlling symptoms without systemic effects or seriously suppressing hypothalamic-pituitary-adrenal cortex functions (Harris 1975, Miyamoto et al 1975).

Systemic lupus erythematosus is not uncommon in women in the child-bearing age group and the beneficial effects of corticosteroids are dramatic (Garsenstein et al 1962). Patients with systemic lupus erythematosus should have plasma deoxyribonucleic acid (DNA) antibody and complement ($C_3$ and $C_4$) levels estimated serially during pregnancy and the dose of steroids increased if either clinical manifestations or changes in DNA antibody or complement levels suggest increased disease activity. Exacerbation of lupus in the puerperium may be controlled by increasing the dose of steroids (Grigor et al 1977).

Corticosteroids are used in patients with inflammatory bowel disease such as ulcerative colitis and regional enteritis (Crohn's disease). There is an increased incidence of relapse in the puerperium which responds to steroid therapy. A severe attack of ulcerative colitis can often be managed with prednisolone enemas.

Renal transplant patients are usually taking corticosteroids with azathioprine for immunosuppression. Pregnancy is relatively uncomplicated and in a recent report by the European Dialysis and Transplant Association (1980) among 110 babies born to transplant recipients, there were only 3 major and 2 minor developmental anomalies. Rejection episodes should be treated by appropriate doses of steroids.

Herpes gestationis is a rare autoimmune disease with an incidence of 1 in 4500 pregnancies and the only effective treatment is systemic corticosteroids (Russell 1962).

Long term use of corticosteroids suppresses ACTH secretion and administration of doses exceeding the equivalent of the physiological secretion of 25 mg of cortisone daily also produces direct suppression of the adrenal cortex. For many months after treatment is discontinued there is a risk of circulatory collapse in patients subjected to surgery (Bayliss 1958) or of postpartum collapse at a confinement. In practice it is safer to assume that any patient who has received steroids within the previous 12 months may have deficient adrenal response to stress. These patients need routine steroid cover with severe illness, general anaesthesia, a surgical procedure or a confinement.

*Acute complications of pregnancy*

Dewhurst (1951) reported four cases of adrenal gland haemorrhage in pregnancy in patients with unexplained collapse, and stressed the importance of considering this possibility in a collapsed patient whose diagnosis remains obscure and who fails to respond to the usual supportive measures. Hydrocortisone should be given intravenously.

In the United States of America considerable use has been made of massive doses of steroids in the management of bacteriogenic shock due to Gram negative infection (Schumer and Nyhus 1970, Schumer 1976). The drugs improve cardiac output and act as peripheral vasodilators permitting more fluid infusion. In a combined prospective and a retrospective trial it was shown that the overall mortality was significantly less in the steroid group than in the control group (Schumer 1976).

*Premature labour*

Respiratory distress syndrome is a lethal disease and is still the commonest cause of death in preterm infants. The advantage of giving steroids to the mother to reduce the chance of respiratory distress is greatest in preterm labour at between 28 and 32 weeks maturity but a few babies up to 34 weeks may be benefited. The steroid effect only persists for 7 to 10 days. Logically, if the patient is still undelivered and of less than 32 weeks maturity, the course of steroids should be repeated weekly. Howie and Liggins (1977) were unable to show any advantage if the dose of betamethasone was doubled from 12 to 24 mg/day.

In view of recent concern about the possible adverse effects of corticosteroids on the developing brain in animals (see Sachs 1981) the treatment is best carried out according to the original protocol of Liggins and Howie (1972). They recommend 12 mg of betamethasone in a 24 hour period and unless delivery has already occurred, a second injection of a similar dose to be given 24 hours later.

Follow-up of babies treated in this way has shown no residual ill-effects (Howie and Liggins 1977).

## Effects on the fetus

### *Animal studies*

The most important feature of the animal work on teratogenic potential of corticosteroids is the very wide species variation (see Tuchman-Duplessis 1975). The mouse is very sensitive to the production of cleft palate—even stimulation of the adrenal glands with ACTH in pregnancy will produce this defect. The mechanism may be the production of oligohydramnios by the steroids, associated with a rigid fetal craniospinal articulation. Rabbits are sensitive, but the malformations produced are mainly cardiac; the anomalies can occur even after topical applications to the conjunctival sac. In addition, in rabbits corticosteroids cause severe intra-uterine growth retardation and often fetal death. In contrast, rats and monkeys are very tolerant of corticosteroids in pregnancy, abnormalities or growth retardation only occurring uncommonly, with high doses of the most potent compounds.

When teratogenic effects are produced, the response varies according to the genetic constitution of the strain of animals, the dose used and the duration of gestation when it is given. Fraser and Fainstat (1951) injected cortisone at different stages of gestation in five genetically different strains of pregnant mice. Doses varying from 0.625 mg to 10 mg/day were used and all mice were treated for 4 days. Treated females of two groups produced relatively more defective offspring than other strains. The incidence of cleft palate in the progeny of these two strains was 79 per cent when the treatment was started in early pregnancy, compared to an incidence of 29 per cent when the steroids were given in late pregnancy. Ten animals were treated with 5 or 10 mg of cortisone per day; in the susceptible strain there was resorption of the litters in most pregnancies and a high incidence of cleft palate in the few litters that survived. Other defects discerned included shortening of the head and spina bifida. In susceptible strains treated with 1.25 mg to 2.5 mg/day of cortisone for 4 days there was marked reduction in birth weight of the offspring. Cleft palate can be produced in rabbits. A parallel experiment performed in pregnant rabbits by injecting cortisone acetate in daily doses of 25 mg and 30 mg for 4 consecutive days showed a high incidence of this defect (Fainstat 1954). The palate is usually closed in the rabbit on the twentieth day of pregnancy and therefore cortisone injections were begun on the fourteenth or fifteenth day of gestation. Seventeen of the 35 embryos had a median post-alveolar cleft palate whereas none of the 36 control embryos had cleft palate. Embryos with cleft palate weighed less and twelve of the 35 embryos were born dead. DeCosta and Abelman (1952) showed high fetal wastage in pregnant rabbits injected with cortisone acetate in daily doses of 15 mg but in only one fetus had the branchial arches failed to fuse in the midline. None of the other animals in which cortisone was injected in early pregnancy had gross congenital defects. Similarly Motoyama et al (1971) reported increased fetal death in rabbits injected with 10 to 30 mg/kg of cortisol for 3 days.

In order to understand the relation of these animal experiments to human therapeutics it is important to appreciate that the doses employed in the animals are equivalent to between 20 and 100 times a 'replacement' dose of steroids for a human patient.

*Human studies*

In the last 30 years steroids have been used to treat many thousands of pregnant women, and there is no very clear evidence of a teratogenic effect of therapeutic doses in humans.

In 1960 Bongiovanni and McPadden made a thorough review of the world literature. Among 260 women who were given pharmacological doses of cortisone or its analogues during pregnancy, there were 1 abortion, 15 premature infants and 8 stillbirths. There were only two babies with cleft palate and one baby presented evidence of adrenocortical failure. No other major malformations were noted. Studies of series of cleft palates reported from the whole population of Great Britain by Oldfield (1949) and Holdsworth (1954) show a control incidence varying from 1 in 600 to 1 in 1000 live births in women not treated with steroids in pregnancy.

Propert (1962) reported 28 pregnancies in 15 patients with rheumatoid arthritis, systemic lupus erythematosus and ankylosing spondylitis on corticosteroids. Four pregnancies ended in abortion and three in fetal death; one infant had a cleft palate. The birth weights of the term infants were within normal range. Serment et al (1968) accumulated 530 cases from the literature and found an overall congenital malformation rate of 2 per cent, which does not differ from that in control populations. There were two babies with cleft palate and one with hare-lip. These malformations were noticed to be associated with large doses of corticosteroids administered during the first trimester. One baby had adrenal hyperplasia and two had acute adrenal insufficiency (Serment and Ruf 1968, cited by Tuchmann-Duplessis 1975). There have been a few isolated case reports of cleft palate in the babies of women given high doses of glucocorticosteroids in early pregnancy (Harris and Ross 1956). Wells (1953) treated 27 patients with hyperemesis gravidarum with large doses of cortisone. Twenty four normal babies were delivered; there was one baby with coarctation of aorta, one with a club foot and one with undescended testes.

Warrell and Taylor (1968) reported poor pregnancy outcomes in women receiving prednisolone for various medical disorders. Among 34 pregnancies, 9 presented with placental insufficiency and there were 8 stillbirths. On the other hand Yackel et al (1966) were unable to show any increased incidence of low birth weight babies in 20 pregnancies in women on corticosteroids. Brown and Smith (1968) had only two babies with growth retardation among 26 patients treated with cortisone analogues during pregnancy. In Grigor et al's (1977) series of patients with systemic lupus erythematosus, dysmature babies were less common in the patients given corticosteroids than in those not so treated. More recently, Reinisch et al (1978) found an incidence of 13.9 per cent of small-for-dates babies from infertile mothers treated with prednisone, 10 mg daily throughout pregnancy. This was compared to an incidence of 1.5 per cent in a control group, a statistically significant difference. It is difficult to see why the incidence of dysmaturity in the control group was so low, as it should be 10 per cent by definition.

*In summary* there may be a very small risk of cleft palate and intra-uterine growth retardation in the fetus when corticosteroids are taken by women during early pregnancy. As any potential adverse effects are likely to be dose related, it is advisable to give the smallest dose compatible with the control of the mother's disease in the first trimester of pregnancy.

The overall incidence of spontaneous abortion, stillbirth and premature labour is probably not increased by patients taking corticosteroids during pregnancy. It is clear that the disease for which steroids are given is the main factor causing dysmaturity. The hazards of not treating the mothers could be much greater (Scott 1968).

*Neurological and behavioural effects.*

There has been some concern about the potential of steroids given in the third trimester of pregnancy for affecting brain development. An analogy has been drawn between the intra-uterine development of the brain in the human fetus during the third trimester of pregnancy and that in newborn rats (Sachs 1981). Administration of glucocorticoids to neonatal rats affects brain cell division and brain weight is reduced by 30 per cent (Cotterrell et al 1972). In the newborn rat corticosteroids impair brain cell proliferation, produce abnormal electrophysiological response, inhibit development of circardian rhythm, and affect emotional reactivity. Cortisol treated animals have retarded development of sensorimotor mechanisms and delayed motivation for swimming (Schapiro et al 1970). Reduced DNA synthesis following postnatal corticosterone treatment in rats is mainly due to suppression of glial cell multiplication (Howard and Benjamin 1975).

The analogy with the human fetus *in utero* is tenuous. The dose of corticosteroids given to the newborn rats (Cotterrell et al 1972) is equivalent to between 5 and 25 times the dose of betamethasone given to a pregnant woman with the objective of maturing fetal lecithin-sphingomyelin ratio (Crowley, 1981).

*Human studies.* The first 318 children whose mothers were treated with steroids antenatally to prevent respiratory distress syndrome have been followed up to 4 years of age (Howie and Liggins 1977) and to date no adverse effects have been found. Similar studies should be extended up to school age in order to establish the absence of neurological and intellectual sequelae.

Attempts have been made to treat respiratory distress syndrome in the neonatal period by administering corticosteroids. Fitzhardinge et al (1974) treated a group of neonates with respiratory distress syndrome with high doses of intravenous hydrocortisone. At 1 year of age there was no apparent difference in the growth rate between the steroid treated and control babies but there was a slightly increased incidence of abnormal motor function and abnormal electroencephalograms. Postnatal corticosteroid treatment is also associated with an increased incidence of intraventricular haemorrhage.

*Risk of infection*

Corticosteroids suppress the immune system and responsiveness to infection and there is potential risk of infection in mother and the newborn when steroids have been administered antenatally. The risk is increased in the presence of ruptured membranes. Howie and Liggins (1977) did not find any significant increase in the incidence of neonatal infection even when the membranes have been ruptured for more than 24 hours, when the patients were given prophylactic antibiotics.

Wong and Taeusch (1978) found an increased risk of infection with steroid treatment. Taeusch et al (1979) in a prospective trial showed an apparently increased incidence of maternal infection in women treated with corticosteroids when the membranes have been ruptured more than 48 hours but the effect was not statistically significant. Kappy et al (1979) demonstrated no increase in infectious morbidity in the presence of prolonged ruptured membranes but there was an increase in bacterial colonisation of the baby. After steroid treatment, newborn babies should be observed for early signs of infection. When there is history of premature rupture of membranes there is a case for prophylactic antibiotic treatment. If there is any respiratory distress in the newborn, antibiotic treatment should be instituted.

**Maternal risks**

The maternal risk which must be prevented is that of development of a chronic or acute hypo-adrenal state. Patients who have had previous steroid treatment may develop hypotension or hyperemesis in pregnancy and require steroid supplements throughout. Patients taking steroids may develop the same symptoms from inadequate doses; 5 to 7.5 mg of prednisolone daily should be regarded as a maintenance dose in pregnancy. Both groups must have parenteral hydrocortisone supplements to cover labour or surgical procedures.

Women on steroid treatment in pregnancy should be tested regularly for possible long-term complications, such as diabetes mellitus, and treated promptly. If hypertension develops in a pregnant patient taking steroids, it should be presumed to be due to essential hypertension of pregnancy or pre-eclampsia, or to the disease process for which the steroids are being given. Pregnancy hypertension should be treated appropriately; if there is exacerbation of a disease such as systemic lupus erythematosus, the hypertension may respond to an increase in the dose of steroids. We have not seen a case where steroids were responsible for hypertension in pregnancy, in managing over 200 cases over 25 years (Hawkins, personal communication 1981), but if the hypothesis needs to be tested this can be done with a short-term reduction in steroid dose.

Steroids increase calcium excretion and therefore adequate calcium intake should be maintained. The potential for peptic ulceration with steroids is present in pregnancy. The drugs should be taken with meals and antacids prescribed if large doses are used. There is a slightly increased susceptibility to viral and bacterial infection; opportunities for acquiring viruses should be avoided and bacterial infections should be treated promptly with antibiotics.

## CONCLUSION

Apart from the occasional patient with Addison's disease, corticosteroid treatment has made successful pregnancy possible for a variety of patients with medical disorders such as bronchial asthma, systemic lupus erythematosus or a renal transplant. The larger human studies have reported little if any increase in the incidence of cleft palate in spite of world-wide use of steroids for many years. Administration of corticosteroids in premature labour has reduced the incidence and severity of respiratory distress syndrome in preterm babies. Long-term follow-up of infants exposed to corticosteroids *in utero* has so far shown no sequelae with respect to brain development, but such studies are few and further work is indicated.

### REFERENCES


Bayliss R I S 1958 Surgical collapse during and after corticosteroid therapy. British Medical Journal ii: 935–936

Bongiovanni A M, McPadden A J 1960 Steroids during pregnancy and possible fetal consequences. Fertility and Sterility 2: 181–186

Brown J B, Smith M A 1968 Excretion of urinary oestrogens in pregnant patients treated with cortisone and its analogues. Journal of Obstetrics and Gynaecology of the British Commonwealth 75: 819–828

Crowley P 1981 Corticosteroids in pregnancy. The benefits outweigh the costs. Journal of Obstetrics and Gynaecology 1: 147–150

Cotterrell M, Balázs R, Johnson A L 1972 Effects of corticosteroids on the biochemical maturation of rat brain: postnatal cell formation. Journal of Neurochemistry 19: 2151–2167

Dewhurst C J 1951 The syndrome of suprarenal haemorrhage in the adult with a report on four cases in association with pregnancy. British Medical Journal ii: 22–26

DeCosta E J, Abelman M A 1952 Cortisone and pregnancy. An experimental and clinical study of the Effects of Cortisone on gestation. American Journal of Obstetrics and Gynecology 64: 746–767

European Dialysis and Transplant Association 1980 Successful pregnancies in women treated by dialysis and kidney transplantation. British Journal of Obstetrics and Gynaecology 87: 839–845

Fainstat T 1954 Cortisone-induced congenital cleft palate in Rabbits. Endocrinology 55: 502–508

Fitzhardinge P M, Eisen A, Letjenyi C, Metrakos K, Ramsay M 1974 Sequelae of early steroid administration to the newborn infant. Pediatrics 53: 877–883

Fraser F C, Fainstat T D 1951 Production of congenital defects in the offspring of pregnant mice treated with cortisone. Pediatrics 8: 527–533
Garsenstein M, Pollak V E, Kark R M 1962 Systemic lupus erythematosus and pregnancy. New England Journal of Medicine 267: 165–169
Graber A L, Ney R L, Nicholson W E, Island D P, Liddle G W (1965). Natural history of pituitary-adrenal recovery following long term suppression with corticosteroids. Journal of Clinical Endocrinology and Metabolism 25: 11–16
Grigor R R, Shervington P C, Hughes G R V, Hawkins D F 1977 Outcome in pregnancy in systemic lupus erythematosus. Proceedings of the Royal Society of Medicine 70: 99–100
Harris D M 1975 Some properties of beclomethasone dipropionate related steroids in man. Postgraduate Medical Journal (Supplement 4) 51: 20–25
Harris J W S, Ross I P 1956 Cortisone therapy in early pregnancy: Relation to cleft palate. Lancet i: 1045–1047
Holdsworth W G 1954 Early Treatment of cleft-lip and cleft-palate. British Medical Journal i: 304–308
Howard E, Benjamin S J A 1975 DNA ganglioside and sulfatide in brains of rats given corticosterone in infancy, with an estimate of cell loss during development. Brain Research 92: 73–87
Howie R N, Liggins G C 1977 Clinical trial of antepartum betamethasone therapy for prevention of respiratory distress in preterm infants. Anderson A, Beard R, Brudenell J M, Dunn P M (editors) In: Pre-term labour. Proceedings of the Fifth Study Group of the Royal College of Obstetricians and Gynaecologists. Royal College of Obstetricians and Gynaecologists, London, pp. 281–289
Kappy K A, Cetrulo C L, Knuppel R A, Ingardia C J, Sbarra A J, Scerbo J C, Mitchell G W 1979 Premature rupture of the membranes: a conservative approach. American Journal of Obstetrics and Gynecology 134: 655–661
Liggins G C, Howie R N 1972 A controlled trial of antepartum glucocorticoid treatment for prevention of the respiratory distress syndrome in premature infants. Pediatrics 50: 515–525
Livanou T, Ferriman D, James V H T 1967 Recovery of hypothalamo-pituitary adrenal function after corticosteroid therapy. Lancet ii: 856–859
Miyamoto T, Osawa N, Makino S, Horiuchi Y 1975 Effect of beclomethasone dipropionate inhalation on adrenal function. Postgraduate Medical Journal 51: 25–26
Motoyama E K, Orzaiesi M M, Kikkawa Y, Kaibara M, Wu B, Zigas C J, Cook C D 1971 Effect of cortisol on the maturation of fetal rabbit lungs. Pediatrics 48: 547–555
Oldfield M C 1949 Modern trends in hare-lip and cleft palate surgery. With a review of 500 cases. British Journal of Surgery 37: 178–194
Propert A J 1962 Pregnancy and adrenocortical hormones. British Medical Journal i: 967–972
Reinisch J M, Simon N G, Karon W G, Gandelman R 1978 Prenatal exposure to prednisone in humans and animals retards intrauterine growth. Science 202: 436–438
Russell B 1962 Herpes gestationis. Proceedings of the Royal Society of Medicine 55: 464
Sachs B P 1982 Corticosteroids in pregnancy. Their potential hazards and track record. Journal of Obstetrics and Gynaecology 1: 143–146
Schapiro S, Salas M, Vukovich K 1970 Hormonal effect on ontogeny of swimming ability in the rat: assessment of central nervous development. Science 168: 147–151
Schumer W 1976 Steroids in the treatment of clinical septic shock. Annals of Surgery 184: 333–341
Schumer W, Nyhus L M (editors) 1970 Corticosteroids in the treatment of shock. University of Illinois Press, Chicago and London

Scott J K 1968 Fetal risk with maternal prednisolone. Lancet i: 208
Serment H, Charpin J, Tessier G, Felce A 1968 Corticothérapie et grossesse. Bulletin de la Fédération des Societés de gynécologie et d'obstétrique de langue française 20: 159–161
Sidhu R K, Hawkins D F 1981 Corticosteroids. In: Wood S M, Beeley L (editors) Prescribing in pregnancy. Clinics in Obstetrics and Gynaecology 8(2). Saunders. London, pp 383–404
Taeusch H W, Frigoletto F, Kitzmiller J, Avery M E, Hehre A, Forum B, Lawson E, Neff R K 1979 Risk of respiratory distress syndrome after prenatal dexamethasone treatment. Pediatrics 63: 64–72
Tuchmann-Duplessis H 1975 Drug effects on the fetus. A survey of the mechanisms and effects of drugs on embryogenesis and fetogenesis. Adis Press, New York, pp. 219–221
Warrell D W, Taylor R 1968 Outcome for the fetus of mothers receiving prednisolone during pregnancy. Lancet i: 117–118
Wells C N 1953 Treatment of hyperemesis gravidarum with cortisone. American Journal of Obstetrics and Gynecology 66: 598–601
Wong Y L, Taeusch H W 1978 White blood cell changes and incidence of fever after maternal treatment with glucocorticoids. Pediatric Research 12: 501
Yackel D B, Kempers R D, McConahey W M 1966 Adrenocorticosteroid therapy in pregnancy. American Journal of Obstetrics and Gynecology 96: 985–989

# 11

P.J. Bolton

# Drugs of abuse

## I SMOKING IN PREGNANCY

The incidence of smoking in pregnancy has been reported as ranging from 17 per cent in France to 50 per cent in the United States of America (see Pirani 1978, for review). In Great Britain one report shows that 40 per cent of women smoked before pregnancy but this incidence fell to 27 per cent after 16 weeks (Butler and Alberman 1969). Chewing tobacco is also quite common in some countries. In one Indian community 16.5 per cent of pregnant women chewed tobacco (Krishna 1978). Whichever way tobacco is taken it represents a risk to the developing fetus.

### EFFECTS OF SMOKING ON PREGNANCY AND THE FETUS

#### Spontaneous abortions

It has been suggested that the incidence of spontaneous abortions among smokers is somewhat increased compared with that in non-smokers (Zabriskie 1963, O'Lane 1963), the difference found being between 12 and 8 per cent respectively. It is difficult to assess the significance of these findings as many abortions remain unreported and there are other variables which affect spontaneous abortion.

#### Congenital abnormalities

There does not appear to be an increase in congenital malformations associated with cigarette smoking, with the possible exception of neural tube defects, where there may be a very small increase in smokers in social classes I and II (Evans et al 1979).

#### Placental changes

As pregnancy advances in heavy smokers the placenta may develop histopathological changes (Asmussen 1977, Naeye 1978), including broadening of the basement membrane of the placental villi, intimal damage of the placental vessels, and increase in the collagen content of the villi. These changes are characteristic of underperfusion from the uterus, which is probably intermittent rather than continuous because the smoker's decidua has few of the arterial changes associated with chronic underperfusion. Lehtovirta and Forss (1978) estimated intervillous placental blood flow using $^{133}$Xe and demonstrated an acute decrease associated with cigarette smoking, which disappeared within 5 minutes. These acute and chronic changes could be responsible for a decrease in placental oxygen transfer.

**Premature labour**

The incidence of both low birth weight infants (less than 2500 g) and preterm deliveries before 37 weeks is higher in mothers who smoke during pregnancy (Pirani 1978).

**Fetal growth and maternal weight gain**

Many authors have found a small decrease in the average size of babies born to mothers who smoke during pregnancy. Growth retardation can be assessed with antenatal ultrasonic biparietal diameter measurements, which show a rather lower average rate of increase in some women who smoke. This decrease in growth may be seen from 21 weeks onwards (Murphy et al 1980). There is disagreement about the relation of this association of maternal weight gain and calorie intake. Rush (1974) and Davies et al (1976) found that poor maternal weight gain during pregnancy in women who smoked was associated with a greater degree of intra-uterine growth retardation. Intra-uterine growth retardation did not occur in their series if maternal weight gain was normal. Meyer (1978) found maternal weight gain distributions to be the same for smokers and non-smokers. These observations are consistent with the view that poor weight gain in maternal smokers is merely symptomatic of intra-uterine growth retardation (Elder et al 1970), rather than a direct consequence of smoking.

Examples of the decrease in birth weight are summarised in Table 11.1. Mothers who smoke in one pregnancy and not in another have smaller babies in the pregnancies in which they smoke irrespective of the birth order (Naeye 1978).

Hormone assays on plasma and urine may be used to assess fetal wellbeing as they merely reflect the status of the feto-placental unit, and do not seem to be specifically associated with smoking. Lee et al (1980) studied placental lactogen levels in a large series of patients and found no difference between the levels found in smokers and non-smokers who delivered babies of comparable weights.

**Table 11.1** Mean birth weights at various gestations in smokers and non-smokers (Naeye 1978)

| Maturity (weeks) | Mean birth weight (g) | | |
|---|---|---|---|
| | Non-smokers | Cigarettes/day | |
| | | 1–20 | Over 20 |
| 31 | 2624 | 2415 | 1887 |
| 34 | 2798 | 2615 | 2488 |
| 37 | 3007 | 2848 | 2816 |
| 40 | 3341 | 3189 | 3188 |
| 43 | 3438 | 3274 | 3346 |

Falls in placental lactogen were seen in patients who delivered babies of low birth weight, merely reflecting the degree of placental insufficiency and intra-uterine growth retardation.

In interpreting information on smoking and fetal dysmaturity to patients, the obstetrician should bear in mind that the data in Table 11.1 are statistical in nature. The reduction in mean birth weights is influenced by a relatively few women with discernible intra-uterine growth retardation, to which other predisposing factors may have contributed. The babies of the majority of even heavy smokers in pregnancy grow normally.

## Fetal breathing

Cigarette smoking has been shown to cause a reduction in the incidence of fetal breathing movements in both normal and abnormal pregnancies (Manning and Feyerabend 1976). This reduction was shown to be related to the rise in maternal plasma nicotine rather than rises in carboxyhaemoglobin.

## Pre-eclampsia

Many authors have found a decrease in the incidence of pre-eclampsia in smokers (Pirani 1978). The reason for this is uncertain but when pre-eclampsia with proteinuria does develop in a smoker the prognosis is poor. The incidence of antepartum haemorrhage is slightly increased in women who smoke (Butler and Alberman 1969) presumably because of reduced blood flow causing ischaemia.

## Perinatal mortality

The estimated perinatal mortality rate for babies of mothers who smoked in pregnancy in 1958 was 41.1/1000 births and for non-smokers 32.0/1000 births in data collected from the British Perinatal Mortality Survey (Butler and Alberman 1969). Both stillbirths and neonatal deaths were estimated by Butler et al (1972) to be 28 per cent higher in smokers. Whilst women who smoked before pregnancy may have a slightly worse prognosis, the relation to perinatal deaths is not nearly so consistent as is the case with consumption during pregnancy (Table 11.2). It appears that the smoking habits which becomes established after 16 weeks are the most important. The increased perinatal mortality is accounted for by prematurity and intra-uterine growth retardation. Butler and Alberman's (1969) study was of a sample equivalent to 150 000 births. Other studies which failed to show an increase in perinatal mortality were smaller and contained a smaller proportion of 'small for gestational age' babies. Butler et al (1972) estimated that on 1970 figures, 1500 babies died as a result of maternal smoking every year in England, Scotland and Wales.

**Table 11.2** Relation of stillbirth and neonatal death rate to the number of cigarettes smoked during pregnancy. (Data from Butler et al 1972.)

| | | Number of cigarettes smoked before pregnancy | | | Total |
|---|---|---|---|---|---|
| | | 0 | 5–9 | 20–30 | |
| Cigarettes/day smoked after 16 weeks | 0 | 32.2* | 31.1 | 35.2 | 32.0 |
| | 1–4 | 39.8 | 38.5 | 43.1 | 38.5 |
| | 5–9 | 44.2 | 42.8 | 47.6 | 42.2 |
| | 20–30 | 40.0 | 39.8 | 43.3 | 41.2 |
| Total | | 32.1 | 39.8 | 43.4 | 34.8 |

* Stillbirths plus neonatal deaths; rate per 1000 births.

Rush and Kass (1972), reviewing 12 388 perinatal deaths and abortions, found the perinatal mortality to be increased by about 34 per cent in smokers. Some of the studies they reviewed failed to show this increased risk but it is difficult to compare different populations. The variation in risk appears greatest among the lower socio-economic groups.

In interpreting this problem to patients, the obstetrician will have at least three reservations. First, the data is presented in a way which has maximum impact as propaganda. A common statement is—for example—that perinatal losses are increased by 30 per cent by smoking in pregnancy (Table 11.3). It would be equally true to comment that the odds against even a possibly 'smoking associated' perinatal loss for a heavy smoker are more than 100 to 1. Second, there is no guarantee if a loss does occur that it could have been prevented if the patient had not smoked—it may have been

**Table 11.3** Risks of smoking (Butler et al 1972)

| | |
|---|---|
| 1. *Prematurity* | |
| Mean gestation reduced by 3 days in smokers | |
| 2. *Growth retardation* | Mean birth weights (*g*) |
| No cigarettes after 16 weeks | 3386 g |
| 20–30 cigarettes after 16 weeks | 3176 g |
| Reduction in mean weight 210 g | |
| 3. *Perinatal mortality (stillbirths and neonatal deaths)* | per 1000 births |
| No cigarettes after 16 weeks | 32.0 |
| 20–30 cigarettes/day after 16 weeks | 41.2 |
| Relative increase in mortality 29 per cent | |

contributed to by factors associated with smoking. Third, the great majority of the data in this field were collected between 10 and 25 years ago, when cigarettes were considerably larger and had a higher nicotine content than they do now. In 1958 the perinatal mortality rate in Great Britain was about 34.9/1000 live births, in 1968 it had fallen to 24.3 and in 1978 to 15.5. As a high proportion of the perinatal lossess in recent years are due to 'unavoidable' causes unrelated to smoking, the real risk of a possibly smoking-associated loss must now be less than the data suggest.

### Long term effects on the child

Some authors suggest that there are no or minimal long-term deleterious effects of smoking during pregnancy. Russell et al (1968) found some recovery of the decreased average weight and head circumference in the babies of smokers until the age of 1 year. This recovery was not complete and some of these babies remained smaller than those of non-smokers. Children of mothers who smoke during pregnancy have, on average, some delay in development (for example, four months for reading and five months for mathematics) at the age of 10 years (Butler and Goldstein 1973).

## POSSIBLE MECHANISMS OF ACTION

Tobacco smoke is a mixture of gases and particulate matter. Although many hundreds of compounds have been identified, the gases carbon monoxide and hydrocyanic acid, and nicotine, are those which have been studied in greatest detail. The actions of these compounds are complex and often antagonistic. Particulate matter may contribute to minor bronchitic changes which may impair maternal respiratory function.

*Carbon monoxide* combines readily with haemoglobin to form

carboxyhaemoglobin. This results in a shift in the oxygen dissociation curve to the left and tends to reduce tissue oxygenation. Transfer of carbon monoxide to the fetus is directly related to the $P_{CO}$ difference between maternal and fetal circulations and is unaffected by relative blood flows. Carboxyhaemoglobin is also present in the fetus and it has been estimated that a carboxyhaemoglobin concentration of 9 per cent in the fetus represents a 41 per cent reduction in fetal blood flow or in fetal haemoglobin concentration (Longo 1970). Cole et al (1972) showed a mean level of carboxyhaemoglobin of 4.1 per cent in smokers compared with 1.2 per cent in non-smokers. This could cause sustained fetal hypoxia (Quigley et al 1979). Davies et al (1979) found that this raised carboxyhaemoglobin in smokers was compensated for by an increase in the average haemoglobin concentration and so the amount of 'available oxygen' remained the same.

*Cyanide and thiocyanate.* Thiocyanate is a metabolite formed by the detoxication of cyanide. The level of thiocyanate present in maternal and cord blood at delivery is significantly higher if the mother smoked during pregnancy (Andrews 1973). It is not certain that raised thiocyanate levels affect fetal growth, but they probably cause disturbances in vitamin $B_{12}$ metabolism. Thiocyanate causes hypotension and may protect the patient against the hypertensive action of nicotine and is perhaps responsible for the reduction in the incidence of pre-eclampsia.

*Nicotine.* The actions of nicotine are widespread and complex. Catecholamines are released and cause an increase in heart rate and cardiac output, vasoconstriction, a rise in blood pressure, hyperglycaemia and a release of free fatty acids; and affect platelet aggregation and coagulation factors, causing hypercoaguability (Pirani 1978, Quigley et al 1979). This action is rapid and causes alterations in fetal heart rate due to an acute decrease in uterine and placental perfusion (Lehtovirta and Forss 1978). Nicotine given by injection causes similar changes in animals and nicotine from tobacco chewing is equally dangerous.

There is no doubt that the compounds present in cigarette smoke can cause physiological changes in the pregnant woman which might cause a degree of acute or chronic fetal anoxia.

## ADVICE TO PATIENTS

The correct time to influence women to stop smoking is *before* they become pregnant. As a result health resources allocated in relation to smoking in pregnancy would best be devoted to informing nulliparous young women of reproductive age of what is known about the relation between smoking and fetal development.

Health education agencies currently indulge in 'scare' advertising directed at pregnant women, implying that unless they stop smoking their baby's growth will be stunted. This is fundamentally dishonest. In the first place only the babies of a small proportion of women who smoke in pregnancy are at risk, and in the second the evidence that discontinuing smoking will improve the situation of the baby is conflicting. Whilst Butler et al (1972) found that women who discontinued smoking by 16 weeks had an improved prognosis, Donovan (1977) was unable to demonstrate any beneficial effect of intensive anti-smoking advice during pregnancy. What can be said with honesty is that smoking in pregnancy is bad for the mother's general health. In addition the effects on the baby's development seem to be directly related to the amount the mother smokes, and the nicotine and other substances absorbed undoubtedly affect the oxygen supply to the baby and get through to the baby, depressing its normal movements.

All patients should be asked about their smoking habits when first seen in the ante-natal clinic and, if they smoke, informed of the potential ill-effects on the fetus. Many will be able to reduce or stop smoking, particularly if they have some nausea in early pregnancy. Chewing gum which contains nicotine is not a safe alternative, as nicotine is one of the more dangerous constituents of cigarettes. 'Smoking cures' containing quinine and similar substances may well do more harm than the smoking itself. Hypnosis is sometimes effective in pregnant patients who desire to stop-smoking but seem unable to succeed in their objective.

If the patient continues to smoke the pregnancy should be carefully monitored for signs of intra-uterine growth retardation. Davies et al (1979) showed that if smoking is stopped for only 48 hours there is a significant rise of 8 per cent in available oxygen from the maternal blood. This may be very important in late pregnancy. All patients who are to be delivered electively, especially by caesarean section, should be discouraged from smoking for several days before delivery.

## CONCLUSION

Smoking represents a genuine statistical risk to pregnancy (Table 11.3) with a demonstrable physical background. That this risk appears small to individual patients should not be allowed to induce a false sense of security. Intensive advice given during pregnancy has given disappointing results. The prognosis for the babies of patients subjected to such programmes is not improved. Education of potential mothers must start before conception.

## II THE FETAL ALCOHOL SYNDROME

It has been known for centuries that alcohol taken in excess in pregnancy may damage the fetus. An increase in perinatal mortality and morbidity was noticed during the English gin epidemic of 1720 to 1750 (Warner and Rosett 1975). During the past few decades more reports have appeared of the adverse effect on fetal growth and development and in 1973 the term 'fetal alcohol syndrome' was coined by Smith and his colleagues in the United States of America (Jones et al 1973). Since then a number of papers have been written pointing out the dangers of consumption of excess alcohol in pregnancy. There is a small but definite risk, but it is unreasonable to allow alarm to develop unnecessarily. The risk should be seen in its correct perspective.

A group of workers in Nantes (Lemoine et al 1968) identified specific dysmorphic features in infants born to alcoholic mothers. They described 127 cases but their paper failed to receive the recognition it deserved. The definitive fetal alcohol syndrome is rare. Jones et al (1973) described the infants of eight unrelated mothers who were drinking large amounts of alcohol. Two required hospitalisation during the pregnancy with delirium tremens, and one was delivered in a drunken stupor. They demonstrated the extreme of a range of abnormalities. The children were small, their mean maturity was 38 weeks and their weight only equivalent to 32 to 34 weeks. None of the infants recovered to normal height and weight for their age even when admitted to hospital with a diagnosis of 'failure to thrive' or when fostered. At one year of age their linear growth rate was only 65 per cent of normal and their average weight 38 per cent of normal. They had microcephaly (head circumference less than the third percentile) and five had cardiac anomalies (ventricular septal defects in three, an atrial septal defect and a patent ductus arteriosus). Subsequently a clear picture of the syndrome emerged.

The four main categories of abnormality found are antenatal growth retardation, a characteristic facial appearance, neurological defects, including mental deficiency, and a tendency to other major anomalies. For a diagnosis of fetal alcohol syndrome at least two of these should be present, including short palpebral fissures or multiple dysmorphic facial features. The facial features are distinctive and help identify the syndrome as an entity. They include a broad flat midface, a broad low nasal bridge, epicanthic folds, short upturned nose, short philtrum, narrow palpebral fissures and frequently facial hirsutism. There may be ear anomalies, large haemangiomata, small nails, altered palmar crease patterns and limited joint movements. Abnormal neurological behaviour is often seen in the neonatal period with irritability, inability to sleep, increased yawning and sneezing and increased head to left preference (Dwyer et al 1978). These features are similar to those seen with narcotic withdrawal and are probably relatively unimportant prognostically. Mental deficiency is the most serious long term consequence of the full syndrome. Some children appear to have minor degrees of the syndrome without the facial features but with some developmental retardation.

## Alcohol intake during pregnancy

It is not known if any particular type of alcoholic drink is more dangerous, although a review of 16 children from France stated that the majority of their mothers were drinking beer (Dehaene et al 1977). Table 11.4 shows the quantities of alcoholic drinks represented by 30 ml of ethanol, an amount which, consumed daily, has been considered to place the fetus at risk. A patient who only drinks socially while pregnant is not likely to be consuming as much as this daily.

**Table 11.4** Quantities of beverages containing 30 ml of ethanol

| | | |
|---|---|---|
| White wine | 300 ml | 2½ wine glasses |
| Red wine | 250 ml | 2 wine glasses |
| Fortified wine | 150 ml | 2 sherry glasses |
| Spirits | 75 ml | 4 measures |
| Beer | 1000 ml | 2 pints |

In a study in Boston (Rosett et al 1978) 13 per cent of mothers interviewed were heavy drinkers with a mean alcohol consumption of 174 ml ethanol daily. Of these, 31 per cent were drinking between 240 and 480 ml of alcohol daily. Their mean consumption of ethanol was estimated at 2.2 g/kg/day. In a unit delivering 2000 women per year in Boston there would thus be 50 patients who drank the equivalent of between almost one and two bottles of spirits per day. In contrast, in a middle and lower social class West London population we were able to identify only two alcoholics among 1000 antenatal patients, and both had decreased their consumption below the risk level during pregnancy.

Evaluating the precise risk of long-term sequelae in the children is difficult. The effects appear to be dose dependent, with a risk of approximately 20 per cent of fetal alcohol syndrome if the intake is in excess of 60 ml of ethanol per day (Hanson et al 1978). These workers, in Seattle, investigated the infants of at-risk mothers. They interviewed 1529 mothers in the fifth month of pregnancy, asking in particular about alcohol, nicotine, drugs and diet. The patients were mainly white, middle-class, well-educated women. They were considered to be at risk if the average daily intake was 30 ml or more of ethanol or if there were episodes of intoxication due to five or more drinks per occasion. On this basis 163 (10.6 per cent) of the mothers were considered to be alcoholics, perhaps by an unduly strict definition. Controls were taken from mild or non-drinking mothers delivered on the same day. The infants of the alcoholic mothers were examined without knowledge of the drinking habits of the mother and classified into three groups: A. abnormal with at least one feature of the fetal alcohol syndrome; B. minor abnormalities, not directly related to the fetal alcohol syndrome; and C. normal (see Tables 11.5, 11.6 and 11.7). Of the 11 babies in group A, two were obvious cases of the syndrome with mothers who were known alcoholics. These were the only two infants with the full fetal alcohol syndrome.

**Table 11.5** Relationship of neonatal abnormality to maternal alcohol intake before recognition of pregnancy (Hanson et al 1978).

| Clinical category | Cases | Average ethanol intake/day | | |
|---|---|---|---|---|
| | | < 3 ml | 3–29 ml | 30 ml or more |
| A. Abnormal with features of fetal alcohol syndrome | 11 | 2 | 0 | 9 |
| B. Minor anomalies | 7 | 2 | 2 | 3 |
| C. Normal | 145 | 58 | 29 | 58 |
| Totals | 163 | 62 | 31 | 70 |

From these results it will be appreciated that abnormal babies are born to a very few mothers with a wide range of drinking habits and that large numbers of heavy drinkers deliver entirely normal babies. Hanson et al (1978) warn of the danger of even small amounts of alcohol in pregnancy, suggesting there is a 10 per cent risk of fetal alcohol syndrome where the mother is consuming 30 to 60 ml of ethanol per day. In this group of mothers it should be noted that

**Table 11.6** Relationship of neonatal abnormalities to maternal alcohol intake during the first 5 months of pregnancy (Hanson et al 1978).

| Clinical category | Cases | Average ethanol intake/day | | |
|---|---|---|---|---|
| | | < 3 ml | 3–29 ml | 30 ml or more |
| A. Abnormal with features of fetal alcohol syndrome | 11 | 4 | 4 | 3 |
| B. Minor anomalies | 7 | 2 | 4 | 1 |
| C. Normal | 145 | 73 | 46 | 26 |
| Total | 163 | 79 | 54 | 30 |

none of the infants had the full fetal alcohol syndrome, but they had less severe abnormalities which were not defined. Long-term studies are needed to determine if these babies suffer any permanent damage.

The high risk of abnormalities in infants of known alcoholic mothers was confirmed in a study of the Collaborative Perinatal Project of the National Institute of Neurologic Disease and Stroke in the United States of America (Jones et al 1974). This was a prospective study of 55 000 pregnant women in twelve centres. From their histories 69 women were considered to be chronic alcoholics, although the amount of alcohol consumed daily was not defined. The children of 23 of these alcoholic women were studied with two controls for each patient. The perinatal mortality rate in the alcoholic mothers was 17 per cent compared with 2 per cent in the control group. Borderline to moderate mental deficiency was recorded in 44 per cent, and 33 per cent had features of the full fetal alcohol syndrome. In contrast, we have not delivered a baby with the full fetal alcohol syndrome at Hammersmith Hospital or Queen Charlotte's Maternity Hospital in ten years, encompassing some 50 000 deliveries

**Table 11.7** Average maternal daily ethanol consumption for infants in each clinical category (Hanson et al 1978).

| Clinical category | Before pregnancy | | First five months of pregnancy | |
|---|---|---|---|---|
| | Mean | Range | Mean | Range |
| A. Abnormal with features of fetal alcohol syndrome | 129 ml | (0–774) | 36 ml | (0–250) |
| B. Minor anomalies | 42 ml | (0–207) | 27 ml | (0–150) |
| C. Normal | 24 ml | (0–258) | 18 ml | (0–78) |

(Hawkins 1981), and fetal alcohol babies are extremely rare in Great Britain.

Dobbing (1974) has drawn attention to two periods when the human brain is especially vunerable because of growth spurts of nervous tissue. These are between 12 and 18 weeks of pregnancy, and during the third trimester, extending into early postnatal life. Neuropathological studies have demonstrated structural abnormalities within the brains of infants exposed to alcohol *in utero*. In one series four brains had similar abnormalities caused by failure or interruption in neuronal and glial migrations. The location of the lesion was not constant and in one case it was in the cerebellum (Clarren et al 1978).

On average, consumption of alcohol is decreased in pregnancy (Little et al 1976). The assumption has been made that a high intake in early pregnancy may be an important aetiological factor. On the other hand it is possible that the fetus is more sensitive to the effects of maternal alcohol consumption later in pregnancy, and this is supported by work (Rosett et al 1978) which shows that by reducing alcohol consumption in late pregnancy the risk of fetal alcohol syndrome is much reduced.

**Effect on fetal growth**

Intra-uterine growth retardation is associated with excessive alcohol intake in pregnancy. Dysmaturity associated with fetal alcohol facial features is well documented in the literature (Lemoine et al 1968, Jones et al 1973, Dehaene et al 1977, Hanson et al 1976) and is clearly associated with consumption of large volumes of alcohol, often by patients who are known to be alcoholic.

Lesser degrees of intra-uterine growth retardation and minor anomalies associated with a lesser degree of alcohol intake are less well documented. Little (1977) investigated 264 patients with singleton pregnancies. Smoking was evenly distributed between the groups of patients. She found that a daily consumption of 30 ml and 60 ml of ethanol led to a reduction in mean birth weight of 91 g and 160 g respectively, compared with controls. In this series only seven (2.7 per cent) of the infants weighed less than 2500 g. It is not known why retarded intra-uterine growth occurs but it may be due to either placental or fetal factors.

The variability of the effects of ethanol on the fetus has been reviewed by Clarren and Smith (1978). Variability is also well illustrated in a case of dizygotic twins, where one was significantly more affected than the other (Christoffel and Salafsky 1975). Although no safe lower limit of alcohol intake in pregnancy has been established it seems likely that there is no significant risk of the baby being affected if the average daily intake is less than 30 ml of ethanol and there are no episodes of intoxication from 'binge drinking'. If the daily intake is between 30 ml and 60 ml of ethanol there is a risk of some degree of intra-uterine growth retardation and minor anomalies in about ten per cent of babies.

If the daily intake is in excess of 60 ml of ethanol then there is a significant risk of some degree of fetal abnormality. It should be remembered that the majority of infants of even women who drink heavily will be normal.

## MECHANISM OF THE FETAL ALCOHOL SYNDROME

The full syndrome is undoubtedly related to alcohol consumption and the relationship appears to be a direct one. Whether the same mechanism causes growth retardation associated with smaller intakes of alcohol is not certain. Experiments on rodents have suggested that large amounts of alcohol given to male rats can cause mutations, intra-uterine deaths and decrease in litter size (Badr and Badr 1975). The effect was obtained with doses of 40 per cent alcohol on three consecutive days by gastric tube before mating. The effects were no longer demonstrable three months after the administration of ethanol. Intra-uterine death and minor abnormalities in mice exposed to ethanol during pregnancy were also demonstrated by Kronick (1976). If this mechanism operated in humans one would expect an increase in early spontaneous abortions and congenital abnormalities in children of alcoholic fathers, but it is difficult to see how the dysmorphic facial features of the fetal alcohol syndrome could result.

Alcohol is known to cross the placenta freely (Waltmann and Iniquez 1972) and is therefore present in the fetus. Ethanol itself or one of its breakdown products may cause the fetal syndrome, or co-existing factors may be involved.

### *Ethanol*

A syndrome similar to that caused in human babies has been induced in rodents with large doses of ethanol (Chernoff 1975). For 30 days before conception and throughout pregnancy two strains of mice were given diets with up to 35 per cent of the calories derived from ethanol. Blood alcohol levels ranged from 0 to 92 mmol/l (0 to 420 mg/100 ml). The mice were killed on the eighteenth day of gestation and the litters examined for skeletal and soft tissue malformations. Abnormalities including deficient ossification, low fetal weight and cardiac and neurological abnormalities were found in litters of mice on high ethanol diets. These abnormalities occured with lower amounts of ethanol in the strain of mice with the lower alcohol dehydrogenase activity.

*Acetaldehyde*

Ethanol is oxidised to acetaldehyde by the hepatic enzyme alcohol dehydrogenase, and then further metabolised by aldehyde dehydrogenase. The ethanol is normally cleared from the bloodstream by the liver at a rate of 2.2 mmol/kg/h (100 mg/kg/h). Alcohol is unique in having a 'zero rate equation', the rate of metabolism being independent of the dose or blood level. The plasma acetaldehyde level does not normally exceed 25 to 30 mmol/l (110 to 132 mg/100 ml).

Veghely and Osztovics (1978) published work on lymphocyte and fibroblast cultures from normal and alcoholic mothers. Significant abnormalities in chromosome function were not noticed with concentrations of 110 mmol/l (500 mg/100 ml) ethanol, equivalent to the human lethal plasma level. Acetaldehyde caused the death of cells and chromosomal aberrations. Studies were also undertaken on patients receiving disulfiram and small amounts of alcohol. Disulfiram blocks the oxidation of alcohol at the acetaldehyde stage and causes an accumulation of acetaldehyde. These workers suggest that a plasma acetaldehyde level of above 40 mmol/l (176 mg/100 ml) may cause abnormalities. Patients who are receiving disulfiram and take alcohol may attain plasma acetaldehyde levels in excess of 400 mmol/l (1.76 g/100 ml). Disulfiram alone causes no abnormalities in cultured cells.

Veghely and Osztovics (1978) also studied acetaldehyde levels in alcoholic women who delivered children with the fetal alcohol syndrome. One mother consumed 8.7 mmol/kg (400 mg/kg) body weight of alcohol whilst on disulfiram and her plasma acetaldehyde level rose to 140 mmol/l (616 mg/100 ml). Another mother consumed minimal amounts of alcohol whilst taking disulfiram but had a child with fetal alcohol syndrome. Large doses of metronidazole have similar effects to disulfiram and if the former drug is given in pregnancy the patient should be told to avoid alcohol. The risk, if it exists, is small as the duration of exposure is usually short and metronidazole therapy is avoided in early pregnancy unless really necessary, as a matter of general principle.

There may be other causes for a raised acetaldehyde level in maternal blood after alcohol consumption. In some rat and mouse strains defects in aldehyde dehydrogenase have been found (Koivula et al 1975). This defect may be inherited or acquired, as in alcoholics with clinical or subclinical liver disease. Most mothers who deliver children with the full fetal alcohol syndrome are known alcoholics, but there does not seem to have been any investigation of liver function or blood chemistry in mothers who drink alcohol in pregnancy and deliver growth-retarded but otherwise normal fetuses. Studies on biochemical changes in pregnant alcoholics are needed, and in particular the relation between plasma acetaldehyde levels and the risk of fetal abnormality or growth retardation requires study. If acetaldehyde is the causal agent it should be possible to screen an at-risk population and offer treatment to those patients with an acetaldehyde concentration above the toxic level. These might include patients with only moderate alcohol consumption but with an enzyme defect.

*Vitamin B deficiency*

Many alcoholics are deficient in B vitamins, although in many of the studies both the drinking and non-drinking populations had dietary deficiencies. Growth retardation has been found in populations with gross malnutrition (Smith 1947) but the dysmorphic features characteristic of fetal alcohol syndrome did not occur.

*Amino acid deficiency*

Vitamin and other deficiencies in the diet may cause congenital abnormalities (Smithells et al 1980) and some severe alcoholics are at risk from such deficiencies. These patients are also at risk for intra-uterine growth retardation but there is no evidence that other populations with dietary deficiencies have children with the facial dysmorphic features of fetal alcohol syndrome.

At present the exact aetiology of the fetal alcohol syndrome is unknown. It seems likely the cause is a direct toxic effect but other factors associated with alcoholism may play a part.

## PREVENTION AND MANAGEMENT

Some groups are so worried about the risks of alcohol in pregnancy that they would advocate complete abstinence for all pregnant women. To go to this extreme is unnecessary and impractical. Patients with a modest intake, such as those who are occasional social drinkers, should be firmly reassured, if they inquire, that one or two drinks per day carries a negligible risk. The risk may be less than from some sedatives and tranquillisers. Public health authorities should remember the small size of the problem in this country before undertaking widespread publicity. The pregnant woman has enough to worry about without being burdened with worry and possible guilt about negligible risks.

More important is the identification of women at risk. The number of pregnant alcoholics in Great Britain is small, probably considerably less than 1 per cent. When first seen in the antenatal clinic all pregnant women should be asked about their alcohol intake. Most patients are willing to give a reasonable history of their consumption and whether this has changed since they had become pregnant. If the intake appears high a more detailed history can be obtained by the obstetrician.

There is a tendency for women to reduce their alcohol consumption normally in pregnancy (Little et al 1976), and there is no doubt that alcoholic patients should be offered counselling and support in pregnancy. Many will be able to reduce their alcohol intake greatly.

*Reduction in intake and its effects*

Prison provides one of the few circumstances where alcohol intake can be abolished and William Sullivan, a prison medical officer, observed that several alcoholic women who had had a number of infants with severe and often fatal complications delivered healthy babies while in prison (Sullivan 1899). One can only hope that these women conceived before being imprisoned, and therefore their abstinence occurred at some later stage in the pregnancy. Although it would be ideal for women at risk to stop or reduce drinking before becoming pregnant, Sullivan's findings suggest that there is benefit to be gained by treating the alcoholic later in pregnancy.

Rosett and his co-workers (1978) in Boston set out to prove the benefits of treatment. In their antenatal clinics 9 per cent of the patients were heavy drinkers and in these women there was an incidence of congenital anomalies, growth retardation and functional abnormalities twice that of moderate or non-drinkers. Patients who drank heavily were encouraged to participate in a treatment programme. This included education about the risks of alcohol and support in their attempt to reduce consumption. Counselling, usually on an individual basis, took place on the same days as the antenatal clinic visits. Fifteen patients were able to reduce or stop drinking. The results are impressive (Table 11.8). Those patients who participated in the programme were more likely to look after their health in other ways and had received improved care because they attended antenatal clinics regularly. All women at risk should receive expert antenatal care with monitoring of intra-uterine fetal growth.

**Table 11.8** Relation between change in alcohol consumption during pregnancy and offspring (Rosett et al 1978).

| | No change ($n$ = 27) % | Abstained or reduced intake ($n$ = 15) % |
|---|---|---|
| Normal | 7 | 67 |
| Congenital anomalies | | |
| major | 15 | 7 |
| minor | 26 | 0 |
| Premature | 26 | 0 |
| Postmature | 11 | 27 |
| Small for gestational age | 37 | 0 |
| Newborn head below 10th centile | 33 | 0 |
| Newborn length below 10th centile | 15 | 0 |

*Termination of pregnancy*

This has a very limited place in the prevention of fetal alcohol syndrome. There are very few patients in whom alcohol consumption can confidently be predicted to cause long term fetal damage, provided the patient is prepared to reduce her alcohol consumption and attend for regular antenatal care. In patients with severe liver disease associated with alcohol there are often strong socio-economic factors and these would prove a more relevant indication for termination of the pregnancies. Certainly where the alcoholic patient wishes to continue with the pregnancy she should be reassured of the likelihood that her child will be normal if she reduces her alcohol intake.

*Psychiatric support*

Pregnancy provides an excellent opportunity to offer psychiatric support and treatment as there is good motivation on the part of most patients. In units treating large numbers of women at risk the success rate has improved as those providing the treatment at all levels have realised that the problem can be recognised from careful history taking and that therapy is effective. The patients are reassured by this optimism and soon learn of other patients who have benefited (Rosett et al 1977). The treatment includes education about the effects of alcohol and normal reproductive function. Support is given to the patient and she is helped to understand her relationships with friends, society and her child.

*Dietary and vitamin supplements*

The patient's general health should be assessed and investigations performed, including liver function tests and possibly plasma amino acids. Where there are abnormalities specific treatment may be offered. All pregnant alcoholic women should be given dietary advice and adequate protein and general vitamin intake assured, using dietary supplements when necessary. Vitamin B supplements are quite harmless and may well be beneficial. Folic acid, 5 mg daily and strong Vitamin B Compound tablets, B.P.C. or an equivalent preparation should be prescribed, starting as early as possible in the pregnancy. Known alcoholics who intend to have a baby should start this regimen even before conception occurs.

Only when more is known of the mechanisms of the abnormalities will we be able to investigate 'at risk' populations and offer further advice. Until then, advice to patients with low alcohol intake should not be alarmist, encouraging them merely to be sensible. Alcohol consumption is increasing but the amounts taken by pregnant women in Great Britain remains small. Although there are exceptionally few cases of fetal alcohol syndrome, obstetricians and paediatricians must be aware of its existence. They should retain a sense of proportion; it is a rare syndrome usually associated with a very large consumption of alcohol in patients already known to be alcoholic.

## III DRUGS OF ADDICTION IN PREGNANCY

Drug addiction in pregnancy is a major problem in the United States of America. In Great Britain it is much less common, but does represent a risk to the fetus. Reports of the effects on the fetus of addiction to narcotics were rare until the late 1950s although Happel described 12 cases in 1892.

Drug addicts are a difficult group to study as they often receive little or no antenatal care, their diets are deficient in calories, protein and vitamins and they often have co-existing diseases, including virus infections such as hepatitis.

Heroin was widely used to obtain oblivion but its use has declined because of escalating costs and inconsistent quality. Lysergic acid diethylamide (LSD) was used as a hallucinogenic, but its popularity waned with the occurrence of psychoses. Patients now more commonly use several different agents, including narcotics, LSD, cannabis and 'glue' (the organic solvents are the active agents). It is consequently difficult to identify possible causal agents when an abnormality does occur. Drug addicts tend to have a greater than average alcohol consumption before becoming addicted and their intake is as great once they are addicted and pregnant.

Some patients need alcohol detoxification as well as treatment for their drug addiction (Blinick et al 1976).

Infertility is not a general problem with drug addicts but some drugs do reduce fertility. Heroin acts on the hypothalamus leading to depression in the release of gonadotrophins. Gaulder et al (1964) found that 64 per cent of patients on heroin had abnormal menstrual cycles, usually oligomenorrhoea or amenorrhoea. When taking heroin alone the incidence was 73.5 per cent, but if the patients were also taking amphetamines or cannabis it fell to 29 per cent. Heroin either depresses areas within the hypothalamus or blocks transmission of impulses between the basal tuberal region of the adenohypophysis and the median eminence of the hypothalamus. This prevents the release of neuro-humoral substances into the hypophyseal-portal circulation and hence the anterior pituitary gland. Cyclical release of gonadotrophins is inhibited. Amphetamines or cannabis have an opposing stimulatory effect on the hypothalamus. In 10 per cent of these patients there was considerable delay in return to normal menstruation.

Multiple ovulation and multiple pregnancy appear to be common among drug addicts (Rementería and Lotongkhum 1977).

## Narcotics

*Chromosomal aberrations and congenital abnormalities*. The demonstration of a high incidence of minor chromosomal aberrations in mother and baby has little relevance to clinical practice unless it can be correlated with an increase in clinical abnormalities. This is especially the case when chromosome abnormalities are detected with *in vitro* culture techniques. Amarose and Norusis (1976) found that 10 per cent of maternal and infant leucocytes showed chromosomal changes in drug addicts receiving heroin and methadone. These were random and of the acentric fragment type, affecting all chromosomes. There was no relation to drug dose and they were not associated with clinical or pathological syndromes.

Ostrea and Chavez (1979) found 20 major abnormalities in 803 patients taking narcotics during pregnancy and suggested that this incidence was increased. Abuse of other drugs was common in their groups and the incidence of abnormalities in their control group was exceptionally low. The abnormalities were very varied in character. A review of the literature has shown an incidence of congenital abnormalities among drug addicts (the majority on heroin) of between 2.7 and 3.2 per cent, which is in the high normal range. There was an impression of an increased rate of chromosomal abnormalities (Rementería and Lotongkhum 1977). This incidence may not be meaningful, as these patients have many other adverse factors affecting their reproductive function.

Much of the evidence in humans and animals is conflicting (Van Blerk et al 1980). No congenital abnormalities have been associated with the use of methadone.

*Fetal growth and placental insufficiency.* Drug addicts who are not under medical supervision have an increased incidence of low birth weight babies. Fraser (1976) observed that intra-uterine growth retardation occurred in 26 per cent; with good antenatal care the figure was 20 per cent. Blinick et al (1976) found that 29 per cent of infants weighed less than 2500 g (compared with 11 per cent in controls) with only a small contribution from prematurity. Small infant size appears to be associated directly with the drugs taken, rather than the lack of antenatal care. In one series patients who took drugs during pregnancy and had no antenatal care had a higher incidence of intra-uterine growth retardation, 47 per cent, than non-drug takers who failed to attend for antenatal care, 20 per cent, (Connaughton et al 1977).

Post mortem studies have shown this retardation in fetal size to be due to a reduced cell number, with all organs being affected (Naeye et al 1973). A direct effect of heroin on antenatal growth seems likely, as similar effects can be seen in animal experiments. The reduction is not fully explained by reduced maternal food intake.

Meconium staining of the amniotic fluid is common in drug addicts (Blinick et al 1976). Up to 60 per cent of placental specimens from drug addicts show meconium histiocytes, suggesting the occurrence of fetal distress before the onset of labour. This suggests that episodes of acute placental insufficiency occur during late pregnancy.

*Perinatal mortality.* There is an increase in perinatal mortality among drug addicts, mainly associated with low birth weight infants. Stillbirths are not more common in drug addicts who are receiving maintenance treatment, but if they continue to abuse drugs

**Table 11.9** Incidence of perinatal deaths associated with drug abuse (from Rementeria and Lotongkhum 1977). All figures are percentages.

| | Controls | Addicts | | |
|---|---|---|---|---|
| | | No narcotics | Narcotics | All |
| Spontaneous abortions | 5.8 | 8.1 | 12.1 | 10.2 |
| Stillbirths | 1.1 | 1.8 | 1.6 | 1.7 |
| Neonatal deaths | 0.6 | 1.5 | 4.1 | 2.8 |
| Perinatal deaths | 1.8 | 3.1 | 5.1 | 4.2 |
| Infant deaths | 0 | 3.0 | 0.9 | 1.9 |

the incidence rises to 65 to 70 per 1000 births (Rementeria and Nunag 1973). The increase in perinatal deaths is mainly among neonates (Table 11.9) and is greatest when narcotics are taken during pregnancy.

*Effects of drug withdrawal on the fetus*

*Antenatal.* Withdrawal of opiates in late pregnancy can cause uterine irritability leading in some patients to premature labour (Connaughton et al 1977). In the United States of America methadone was restricted by the Food and Drug Administration in 1973 to use for only 21 days, once pregnancy was diagnosed. This edict was rescinded following a report of an intra-uterine death apparently attributable to withdrawal. Fetal death has also been recorded in association with a maternal and fetal withdrawal syndrome in a patient on heroin (Rementeria and Nunag 1973). Zuspan et al (1975) studied serial amniotic fluid adrenaline and noradrenaline levels and found an increase in the level of both amines following a decrease in maternal methadone dose. This was considered to reflect fetal stress and the methadone dose was then increased, with a consequent fall in the amniotic fluid catechol amine levels. These authors suggested that complete drug withdrawal is dangerous in late pregnancy and this view has been reinforced by other workers.

*Postnatal.* Babies with narcotic withdrawal symptoms appear normal at birth but after 24 to 72 hours become progressively restless and irritable. Feeding is poor, diarrhoea is common and the baby may die with convulsions. The mortality is then in excess of 90 per cent if the baby is untreated (Goodfriend et al 1956). Originally treatment was with narcotics and included the mother blowing opium smoke over the baby's face or into its mouth. The use of barbiturates was superseded by that of diazepam ten years ago (Nathenson et al 1971). Fifty per cent of babies of narcotic addicts require diazepam and they should remain in hospital for 14 days, unless asymptomatic and gaining weight. In 10 per cent of babies the onset of withdrawal symptoms will be delayed for 10 to 36 days and if these are not recognised the consequences may be fatal (Kandall and Gartner 1974). There is thus a case for keeping the baby in hospital for observation until progress is satisfactory. The risk is greatest when the problem of drug abuse remains undetected.

*Drug treatment in pregnancy*

The objective in antenatal care is not primarily to stop drug use but to stabilise the dose and where possible to control the patient on methadone. Methadone detoxification programmes in pregnancy have met with little success as almost all patients return to heroin use later in the pregnancy and require repeated admissions to hospital (Blinick et al 1976). More success is obtained with methadone maintenance programmes, although many patients will desire 'kicks' from alcohol, barbiturates and occasionally heroin.

*Management in labour*

Regional analgesia should be used where possible, avoiding narcotics, but methadone may be used where necessary to treat withdrawal symptoms. The incidence of caesarean section is not increased but when the operation is performed the indication is more commonly fetal distress (Ostrea and Chavez 1979). Fetal distress is more common when antenatal control of drug dose is inadequate (Stimmel and Adamson 1976).

*Long term effects on the infant*

There are few long term ill effects on the baby directly attributable to drug abuse in pregnancy (Stimmel and Adamson 1976), although there may be an increase in minor neurological abnormalities where there is intra-uterine growth retardation (Blinick et al 1976). Rementeria and Lotongkhum (1977) have reported an increased incidence of the sudden infant death syndrome. Child abuse is also more common. Where social conditions are adequate subsequent growth of the baby is satisfactory.

**Lysergic acid diethylamide**

Studies on possible adverse effects of LSD in pregnancy are conflicting and inconclusive. Jacobson and Berlin (1972) found that LSD use during pregnancy was associated with a 10 per cent incidence of major congenital anomalies, the majority being neural tube defects. Midline fusion defects were also found in a large percentage of therapeutic abortions in their patients. Fifty per cent of their live-born infants had minor chromosomal abnormalities in the blood at birth but these were no longer detectable by 3 to 6 months. Dumas (1971), studying children offered for adoption, found no significant increase in chromosomal breakage in infancy where the mother had taken LSD during pregnancy. LSD added to cultured human leucocytes will induce chromosomal aberrations, but a similar effect is obtained by adding acetylsalicylic acid (aspirin) to the culture (Jarvik and Kato 1968). Long (1972), reviewing the literature, concluded that there was no firm evidence of teratogenesis of LSD in humans although, noting five cases of limb deficiencies, she urged caution.

Patients receiving LSD therapeutically, and hence as a solitary agent, do not have an increased incidence of low birth weight normal babies (Jacobson and Berlin 1972). Patients who take LSD during pregnancy should be advised to stop taking the drug, but reassured that any potential risks are small. It is reasonable to offer screening for neural tube defects by serum α-fetoprotein estimation and ultrasound.

## Marihuana

Chromosomal aberrations occur when human leucocytes are cultured with marihuana but the incidence is no higher than in control cultures (Neu et al 1969). There is no evidence that marihuana causes congenital abnormalities in humans.

## Other hallucinogens

Abnormalities have been reported with the use of 'angel dust' (phencyclidine) in pregnancy (Golden et al 1980). A baby born to a mother taking 'angel dust' during pregnancy developed abnormal neurological behaviour with lethargy and intermittent hypertonicity. The baby had dysmorphic facial features and developed a spastic quadriplegia. Although this is an isolated report the abnormalities are similar to those observed in animals.

## Amphetamines

Reports have suggested an increased incidence of congenital abnormalities in mothers who take amphetamines during pregnancy. Milkovich and van den Berg (1977) found an excess of oral cleft defects in babies of mothers who received amphetamines during pregnancy. The overall incidence of serious congenital anomalies was no higher than in their control patients. Levin (1971) reported an increased incidence of biliary atresia in infants of mothers receiving amphetamines during pregnancy. This report deserves serious consideration because of the rarity of congenital biliary atresia. In addition, a retrospective study of 184 mothers who delivered babies with congenital heart defects has shown an increased number of women who took amphetamine during their pregnancies (Nova et al 1970). This increase was not confirmed in the more carefully controlled trial of Milkovich and van den Berg (1977). It seems possible that there may be a teratogenic effect associated with the use of amphetamines in early pregnancy and their use as appetite suppressants should be discouraged.

Maternal amphetamine use during pregnancy has also been associated with prematurity, low birth weight and an increased incidence of pre-eclampsia (Eriksson et al 1978). Patients who continue to abuse amphetamines during pregnancy attend antenatal clinics poorly and have a high incidence of hepatitis and gonorrhoea.

There is no evidence from animal work or studies in humans that the appetite suppressant fenfluramine, taken in early pregnancy, is teratogenic. Whilst many doctors disapprove of drugs as an aid to weight reduction, this is still a significant problem. Husbands tend to find a slimmed wife more attractive and pregnancies result.

## CONCLUSION

The prognosis for the infant of a drug-addicted mother is good if she co-operates with antenatal care and drug control. She should be informed of these good results. During pregnancy a woman undergoes a role change to that of a mother and the future of the baby can act as a bribe. The response to sympathetic psychiatric management and perhaps gradual reduction in dose should be rewarding (Goldie 1974). In late pregnancy no attempt should be made to stop narcotics completely; the patient should be maintained on methadone. The newborn should be observed carefully for evidence of narcotic withdrawal symptoms and treated where necessary with diazepam. The baby needs careful supervision for at least 6 weeks. After pregnancy efforts should be made to withdraw the patient from drug use, but results have so far proved disappointing.

### REFERENCES

Amarose A P, Norusis M J 1976 Cytogenetics of methadone-managed and heroin-addicted pregnant women and their newborn infants. American Journal of Obstetrics and Gynecology 124: 635–640

Andrews J 1973 Thiocyanate and smoking in pregnancy. Journal of Obstetrics and Gynaecology of the British Commonwealth 80: 810–814

Asmussen I 1977 Ultrastructure of the human placenta at term. Observations on placentas from newborn children of smoking and non-smoking mothers. Acta obstetricia et gynaecologica Scandinavica 56: 119–126

Badr F M, Badr R S 1975 Induction of dominant lethal mutation in male mice by ethyl alcohol. Nature 253: 134–136

Blinick G, Wallach R C, Jerez E, Ackerman B D 1976 Drug addiction in pregnancy and the neonate. American Journal of Obstetrics and Gynecology 125: 135–142

Butler N R, Alberman E D (editors) 1969 Perinatal problems—the second report of the 1958 British Perinatal Mortality Survey. Livingstone, Edinburgh

Butler N R, Goldstein H 1973 Smoking in pregnancy and subsequent child development. British Medical Journal iv: 573–575

Butler N R, Goldstein H, Ross E M 1972 Cigarette smoking in pregnancy—its influence on birth weight and perinatal mortality. British Medical Journal ii: 127–130

Chernoff G F 1975 A mouse model of the fetal alcohol syndrome. Teratology 11: 14A

Christoffel K K, Salafsky I 1975 Fetal alcohol syndrome in dizygotic twins. Journal of Pediatrics 87: 963–967

Clarren S K, Smith D W 1978 The fetal alcohol syndrome. New England Journal of Medicine 298: 1063–1067

Clarren S K, Alvord E C, Sumi S M, Streissguth A P, Smith D W 1978 Brain malformations related to pre-natal exposure to ethanol. Journal of Pediatrics 92: 64–67

Cole P V, Hawkins L H, Roberts D 1972 Smoking during pregnancy and its effects on the fetus. Journal of Obstetrics and Gynaecology of the British Commonwealth 79: 782–787

Connaughton J F, Reeser D, Shut J, Finnegan L P 1977 Perinatal addiction; outcome and management. American Journal of Obstetrics and Gynecology 129: 679–686

Davies D P, Gray O P, Ellwood P C, Abernathy M 1976 Cigarette smoking in pregnancy; associations with maternal weight gain and fetal growth. Lancet i: 385–387

Davies J M, Latto I P, Jones J G, Veale A, Wardrop C A J 1979 Effects of stopping smoking for 48 hours on oxygen availability from the blood: a study on pregnant women. British Medical Journal ii: 355–356

Dehaene P H, Walbaum A, Titran M 1977 The offspring of chronically alcoholic mothers—a report of 16 cases of fetal alcoholism. Revue française de gynécologie et d'obstétrique 72(7–9): 491

Dobbing J 1974 The later development of the brain and its vulnerability. In: Davis J A, Dobbing J (editors) Scientific foundations of paediatrics. Heinemann, London; Saunders, Philadelphia, pp 565–577

Donovan J W 1977 Randomised controlled trial of anti-smoking advice in pregnancy. British Journal of Preventive and Social Medicine 31: 6–12

Dumas K W 1971 Parental drug usage: effect upon chromosomes of progeny. Pediatrics 47: 1037–1041

Dwyer L S, Keller L S, Streissguth A 1978 Naturalistic observations of newborns: effect of maternal alcohol intake. Alcoholism: Clinical and Experimental Research 2: 171–177

Elder M G, Burton E R, Gordon H, Hawkins D F, Browne J C McC 1970 Maternal weight gain and girth changes in late pregnancy and the diagnosis of placental insufficiency. Journal of Obstetrics and Gynaecology of the British Commonwealth 77: 481–491

Eriksson M, Larsson G, Winbladh B, Zetterström R 1978 The influence of amphetamine addiction on pregnancy and the newborn infant. Acta paediatrica Scandinavica 67: 95–97

Evans D R, Newcome R G, Campbell H 1979 Maternal smoking habits and congenital malformations; a population study. British Medical Journal ii: 171–173

Fraser A C 1976 Drug addiction in pregnancy. Lancet ii: 896–899

Gaulder E C, Littlefield D C, Putoff O E, Seivert A L 1964 Menstrual abnormalities associated with heroin addiction. American Journal of Obstetrics and Gynecology 90: 155–160

Golden N L, Sokol R J, Rubin I L 1980 Angel dust; possible effects on the fetus. Pediatrics 65: 18–20

Goldie L 1974 The role of the psychiatrist in obstetric therapeutics. In: Hawkins D F (editor) Obstetric therapeutics. Baillière Tindall, London, pp 195–198

Goodfriend M J, Shey I A, Klein M D 1956 The effects of maternal narcotic addiction on the newborn. American Journal of Obstetrics and Gynecology 71: 29–36

Hanson J W, Jones K L, Smith D W 1976 Fetal alcohol syndrome, experience with 41 patients. Journal of the American Medical Association 235:1458–1460

Hanson J W, Streissguth A P, Smith D W 1978 The effects of moderate alcohol consumption during pregnancy on fetal growth and morphogenesis. Journal of Pediatrics 92: 457–460

Happel J J 1982 M & S Reporter, Philadelphia, 67: 402. Quoted by Goodfriend et al 1956

Hawkins D F 1981 Effects of drugs in pregnancy and during lactation. In: Roberts D F, Chester R (editors) Changing patterns of conception and fertility. Academic Press, London, pp 135–163

Jacobson C B, Berlin C M 1972 Possible reproductive detriment in L.S.D. users. Journal of the American Medical Association 222: 1367–1373

Jarvik L F, Kato T 1968 Is lysergide a teratogen? Lancet i: 250

Jones K L, Smith D W, Vileland C, Streissguth A P 1973 Pattern of malformation in offspring of chronic alcoholic mothers. Lancet i: 1267–1271

Jones K L, Smith D W, Streissguth A P, Myrianthopoulos N C 1974 Outcome of offspring of chronic alcoholic women. Lancet i: 1076–1078

Kandall S R, Gartner L M 1974 Late presentation of drug withdrawal symptoms in newborns. American Journal of Diseases of Children 127: 58–61

Koivula T, Koivusalo M, Lindros K O 1975 Liver aldehyde and alcohol dehydrogenase activity in rat strains genetically selected for their ethanol preference. Biochemical Pharmacology 24: 1807–1811

Krishna K 1978 Tobacco chewing in pregnancy. Journal of Obstetrics and Gynaecology of the British Commonwealth 85: 726–728

Kronick J B 1976 Teratogenic effects of ethyl alcohol administered to pregnant mice. American Journal of Obstetrics and Gynecology 124: 676–680

Lee J N, Grudzinskas J G, Chard T 1980 Circulating placental lactogen (HPL) levels in relation to smoking during pregnancy. Journal of Obstetrics and Gynaecology 1: 87–89

Lehtovirta P, Forss M 1978 The acute effect of smoking on intervillous blood flow of the placenta. Journal of Obstetrics and Gynaecology of the British Commonwealth 85: 729–731

Lemoine P, Haroussenn H, Borteym J-P, Menuet J-C 1968 Les enfants de parents alcooliques, anomalies observées. A propos de 127 cas. Ouest médical 25: 476–482

Levin J N 1971 Amphetamine ingestion with biliary atresia. Journal of Pediatrics 79: 130–131

Little R E 1977 Moderate alcohol use during pregnancy and decreased infant birth weight. American Journal of Public Health 67: 1154–1156

Little R E, Schultz F A, Mandell W 1976 Drinking during pregnancy. Journal of Studies on Alcohol 37: 375–379

Long S Y 1972 Does L.S.D. induce chromosomal damage and malformations? A review of the literature. Teratology 6: 75–90

Longo L D 1970 Carbon monoxide in the pregnant mother and fetus, and its exchange across the placenta. Annals of the New York Academy of Sciences 174: 313–341

Manning F A, Feyerabend C 1976 Cigarette smoking and fetal breathing movements. British Journal of Obstetrics and Gynaecology 83: 262–270

Meyer M B 1978 How does maternal smoking affect birth weight and maternal weight gain? American Journal of Obstetrics and Gynecology 131: 888–893

Milkovich L, van den Berg B J 1977 Effects of antenatal exposure to anorectic drugs. American Journal of Obstetrics and Gynecology 129: 637–642

Murphy J F, Drumm J E, Mulcahy R, Daly L 1980 The effect of maternal cigarette smoking on fetal birth weight and growth of the fetal biparietal diameter. British Journal of Obstetrics and Gynaecology 87: 462–466

Naeye R L 1978 Effects of maternal cigarette smoking on the fetus and placenta. Journal of Obstetrics and Gynaecology of the British Commonwealth 85: 732–737

Naeye R L, Blanc W, Leblanc W, Khatamee M A 1973 Fetal complications of maternal drug addiction; abnormal growth, infections and episodes of stress. Journal of Pediatrics 83: 1055–1061

Nathenson G, Golden G S, Litt I F 1971 Diazepam in the management of the neonatal narcotic withdrawal syndrome. Pediatrics 48: 523–527

Neu R L, Powers H O, King S, Gardner L I 1969 Cannabis and chromosomes. Lancet i: 675

Nova J J, Vazo T A, Nova A H, Love K E, McNamara D G 1970 Dexamphetamine; a possible environmental trigger in cardiovascular malformations. Lancet i: 1290–1291

O'Lane J M 1963 Some fetal effects of maternal cigarette smoking. Obstetrics and Gynecology 22: 181–184

Ostrea E M, Chavez C J 1979 Perinatal problems (excluding neonatal withdrawal) in maternal drug addiction; a study of 830 cases. Journal of Pediatrics 94: 292–295

Pirani B B K 1978 Smoking during pregnancy. Obstetrical and Gynecological Survey 33: 1–13

Quigley M E, Sheehan K L, Wilkes M M, Yen S S C 1979 Effects of maternal smoking on circulating catecholamine levels and fetal heart rates. American Journal of Obstetrics and Gynecology 133: 685–690

Rementería J L, Nunag N N 1973 Narcotic withdrawal in pregnancy. Stillbirth incidence with a case report. American Journal of Obstetrics and Gynecology 116: 1152–1156

Rementería J L, Lotongkhum L 1977 Drug abuse in pregnancy and neonatal effects. C V Mosby, St Louis

Rosett H L, Ouellette E, Weiner L, Owens E 1977 In: Seixas F A (editor) Currents in alcoholism Vol 1. Grune and Stratton, New York, pp 419–430

Rosett H L, Ouellette E, Weiner L, Owens E 1978 Therapy of heavy drinking during pregnancy. Obstetrics and Gynecology 51: 41–46

Rush D 1974 Examination of the relationship between birth weight, cigarette smoking during pregnancy and maternal weight gain. Journal of Obstetrics and Gynaecology of the British Commonwealth 81: 746–752

Rush D, Kass E H 1972 Maternal smoking: a reassessment of the association with perinatal mortality. American Journal of Epidemiology 96: 183–186

Russell C S, Taylor R, Law C E 1968 Smoking in pregnancy, maternal blood pressure, pregnancy outcome, baby weight and growth and other related factors. A prospective study. British Journal of Preventive and Social Medicine 22: 119–126

Smith C A 1947 Effects of maternal under-nutrition upon the newborn infant in Holland (1944–1945). Journal of Pediatrics 30: 229–243

Smithells R W, Sheppard S, Schorah C J et al 1980 Possible prevention of neural tube defects by preconceptional vitamin supplementation. Lancet i: 339–340

Stimmel B, Adamson K 1976 Narcotic dependency in pregnancy. Methadone maintenance compared to use of street drugs. Journal of the American Medical Association 235: 1121–1124

Sullivan W C 1899 A note on the influence of maternal inebriety on the offspring. Journal of Medical Science 45: 489–503

Van Blerk G A, Majerus T C, Myers R A M 1980 Teratogenic potential of some psychopharmologic drugs: a brief review. International Journal of Gynaecology and Obstetrics 17: 399–402

Veghely P V Osztovics M 1978 The alcohol syndrome, the intrarecombigenic effect of acetaldehyde. Separatum experientia 34: 195

Waltman R, Iniquez E S 1972 Placental transfer of ethanol and its elimination at term. Obstetrics and Gynecology 40: 180–185

Warner R H, Rosett H L 1975 The effect of drinking on offspring: an historical survey of the American and British literature. Journal of Studies on Alcohol 36: 1395–1420

Zabriskie J R 1963 Effect of cigarette smoking during pregnancy. Obstetrics and Gynecology 21: 405–411

Zuspan F P, Gumpel J A, Mejia-Zelaya A, Madden J, Davis R 1975 Fetal stress from methadone withdrawal. American Journal of Obstetrics and Gynecology 122: 43–46

# Premature labour

In the United Kingdom 6.9 per cent of all babies weigh less than 2500 g at birth (Chamberlain et al 1978), but less than one third of these births are due to spontaneous preterm labour (Fedrick and Anderson 1976). The remainder of low birth weight babies include elective preterm deliveries and small-for-dates term infants. In contrast to the results of spontaneous preterm labour, these births have a relatively low perinatal mortality rate (Rush et al 1976). These authors quote an incidence of 3.4 per cent for spontaneous delivery after 22 weeks and before 37 weeks. Fuchs (1976) quoted a higher rate but failed to allow for elective preterm delivery. Data from a computer bank covering 240 274 deliveries indicate that 4.9 per cent of patients delivered infants weighing more than 500 g and less than 2500 g, between 20 and 37 weeks maturity (Kaltreider and Kohl 1980). Elective preterm delivery is included in this data.

While the incidence of preterm labour is low, it is associated with a high perinatal mortality. In the 1958 births survey the perinatal mortality rate was 290 per 1000 for singleton infants born without congenital malformation before 37 weeks and weighing less than 2500 g (Fedrick and Anderson 1976).

Despite the dramatic improvements in neonatal survival reported from specialised centres throughout the 1970s (Stewart et al 1977, Gamsu et al 1979) this relatively uncommon complication of pregnancy makes a major contribution to perinatal mortality. In 1973 and 1974 in the John Radcliffe Hospital, Oxford, spontaneous preterm delivery occurred in 3.4 per cent of total births but accounted for 77.5 per cent of neonatal deaths not associated with congenital abnormality (Rush et al 1976).

In addition to contributing heavily to perinatal mortality, preterm delivery can also lead to mental and physical handicap. Among very small preterm infants weighing less than 1.35 kg at birth and born as recently as the 1960s, up to two-thirds of survivors had severe and permanent mental handicap (Drillien 1972). Only 27.8 per cent of small preterm infants weighing 501 to 1500 g born alive at Hammersmith Hospital in 1961 to 1975 were apparently normal at follow-up (Jones et al 1979). While other authors suggest that increasing survival of very low birth weight infants has been accompanied by a commensurate improvement in the quality of survival, the potential contribution of survivors of preterm birth to the total population of handicapped individuals remains a source of emotive debate (Reynolds and Stewart 1980).

Spontaneous preterm labour also carries serious economic implications. Neonatal intensive care cost approximately £340 per infant per week in 1978 (Hansard 1978). The estimated economic cost of perinatal handicap is currently £373 000 per individual, based on the cost of 40 years stay in a Spastics Society home and 40 years of lost earnings at £5000 per year (House of Commons 1980).

## PREVENTION OF PRETERM LABOUR

The catalogue of mortality, morbidity and economic cost associated with spontaneous preterm birth makes the case for preventing preterm birth self-evident. Attempts to prevent preterm birth have followed two main pathways; the primary prevention of preterm labour and the arrest of preterm labour following its onset. Formalised antenatal scoring systems have been devised to predict the risk of spontaneous preterm birth or low birth weight delivery (Kaminski et al 1973, Kaminski and Papiernik 1974, Fedrick 1976). Low maternal age, low social class, low stature and low body-weight are strikingly associated with preterm labour (Illsley and Thompson 1976). Multiparous women who delivered a preterm infant in the past have a substantially increased risk of repeated preterm birth (Bakketeig and Hoffman 1981). Thus Fedrick's (1976) scoring system can identify a group of multiparae who are at high risk of spontaneous preterm labour, but any intervention aimed at preventing preterm labour in those identified by the scoring system would be applied to twenty women in order to benefit one (Newcombe and Chalmers 1981). Even if intervention of this nature was without risk it would be impractical.

Any antenatal scoring system predicting risk of preterm delivery is only as useful as the measures taken to prevent preterm labour in those it identifies as 'at risk'. Current antenatal care does not even attempt to improve the socio-economic disadvantages which act as significant determinants of preterm labour. Some medical intervention may even increase the psychological stress which seems to be associated with preterm birth (Newton et al 1979).

**General measures**

Primary prevention of preterm labour in all women, but particularly in those at special risk, might include advice to stop smoking before they conceive. A randomised controlled trial has shown that anti-smoking advice given in pregnancy is ineffective. There was an improvement in smoking behaviour but not in perinatal outcome in women intensively and individually counselled at each perinatal visit (Donovan 1977). It has yet to be demonstrated that anti-smoking advice before conception will alter the outcome.

Nutritional supplementation is an appealing possibility in the prevention of preterm birth, in view of the association between preterm birth and low pre-pregnant weight and low socio-economic status (Fedrick and Anderson 1976). In a randomised controlled trial of nutritional supplementation in a poor black community in New York City, length of gestation was increased and the proportion of low birth weight infants reduced in the patients who received a balanced protein calorie complement, consisting of 6 g of animal protein and 322 kcal/day (1352 kJ/day). On the other hand, those who received considerably greater protein supplementation consisting of 40 g of animal protein and 470 kcal/day (1977 kJ/day), were found to have significantly more neonatal deaths than the unsupplemented controls, due to an excess of very early preterm births (Rush et al 1980). This trial, which was criticised as unethical because supplements were withheld from a control group, emphasises the need to test even intervention which seems beneficial, before incorporating it into practice.

While education concerning smoking and balanced nutrition in pregnancy may be offered to all women, only a minority of women need more dramatic intervention such as prolonged periods of bed rest. Women with twin pregnancies represent a high risk group who might benefit from bed rest. The majority of studies on hospital bed rest for patients with twin pregnancies have demonstrated a reduction in preterm labour and low birth weight babies and a lower perinatal mortality (Bender 1952, Browne and Dixon 1963, Jeffrey et al 1973, Laursen 1973, Komáromy and Lampé 1977), though Law (1967) and Weekes et al (1977) failed to show any benefit. The trials have mainly been retrospective studies, and selection of patients may have been biased because twins with better intra-uterine growth are more likely to be diagnosed early. Differences in social class, parity and the readiness of patients to co-operate by accepting hospital admission act as confounding variables. The diagnosis of twin pregnancies by ultrasound should remove the bias introduced by clinical diagnosis and permit a prospective randomised controlled trial of bed rest in twin pregnancies. Meanwhile the implications of Jeffrey et al's (1973) and Komáromy and Lampé's (1977) reports should be noted. Little benefit in terms of a reduction in perinatal mortality from bed rest is found unless delivery before 30 weeks is prevented. If bed rest is considered to be appropriate, it should be initiated between 26 and 30 weeks maturity.

Kass (1960) was the first to emphasise the association between asymptomatic bacteriuria and low birth weight delivery. The nomenclature of the time led to confusion between spontaneous preterm delivery and intra-uterine growth retardation. Kass (1973) was able to report evidence from controlled trials that elimination of bacteriuria reduces morbidity from pyelonephritis in pregnancy and confers a small but significant reduction in the rate of preterm birth. Other authors have failed to show a reduction in preterm delivery in women with treated bacteriuria compared with untreated controls (Gold et al 1966, Robertson et al 1968, Furness et al 1975). Although bacteriuria is unlikely to account for more than 5 to 10 per cent of all cases of spontaneous preterm labour, screening for bacteriuria would appear to be justified (Kass 1973). As screening procedures are relatively inexpensive and the majority of patients respond to a single course of treatment (Brumfitt and Reeves 1968), the entire obstetric population could reasonably be screened. Alternatively, primigravidae, especially those of low socio-economic status, and multiparae with a past history of urinary tract infection in pregnancy, represent suitable populations for screening.

Prospective studies are necessary to evaluate the evidence that coitus in pregnancy precipitates preterm labour in susceptible women (Goodlin et al 1971) or that it increases perinatal morbidity (Naeye 1979). A reasonable approach at present might be to advise against coitus in the late second and early third trimester in women identified by previous history to be at high risk of preterm labour.

While any or all of the measures discussed may reduce the risk of preterm labour in an individual case, the overall incidence of preterm labour appears to be unchanged since 1946 (Chamberlain 1979). The possibility of inhibiting preterm labour by pharmacological methods must be explored.

*Cervical cerclage.* The true incidence of cervical incompetence, its contribution to preterm labour and the ability of cervical cerclage to prevent preterm labour are the subject of considerable debate (Papiernik 1977, Turnbull 1977). The procedure carries a small risk of precipitating intra-uterine infection and abortion, so a scoring system designed to identify those most and least likely to benefit from cervical cerclage might be of value (Dumont and Poizet 1974). A recent retrospective study failed to demonstrate a benefit when cervical cerclage was performed empirically on the basis of two previous mid-trimester abortions or two previous preterm labours (Anderson 1977). A prospective controlled study showed that prophylactic insertion of cervical sutures had no effect on the incidence of preterm labour in twin pregnancies (Weekes et al 1977). While cervical cerclage is of undoubted value in a small number of selected patients, the outcome of the planned Medical Research Council multicentre trial of cervical cerclage may clarify the role of this procedure in more equivocal cases.

## ARREST OF PRETERM LABOUR

Tocolytic drugs may contribute to the management of preterm labour by suppressing uterine contractions for a short time to permit the administration of corticosteroids, or to facilitate the transfer of the patient to a unit with neonatal intensive care facilities. Alternatively, labour might be postponed for several weeks resulting in the birth of a term infant.

A recent summary of recommended management of preterm labour advised the use of tocolytic drugs in spontaneous labour between 26 and 32 weeks of pregnancy, when the cervix is less than 4 cm dilated and the membranes are intact (Ritchie and McClure 1979). Broadly, this describes the practice of 90 per cent of obstetricians in Great Britain (Lewis et al 1980). Treatment with tocolytic agents is often unsuccessful when the membranes have ruptured (Renaud et al 1974). Furthermore, prolongation of pregnancy following spontaneous rupture of the membranes increases the risk of perinatal infection (Eggers et al 1979). Ritchie and McClure's (1979) recommendation to use β-sympathomimetic drugs 'rarely' in the presence of ruptured membranes represents a typical viewpoint. Some authors recommend β-sympathomimetic drugs for 24 hours to permit corticosteroid therapy (British Medical Journal 1979, Creasy and Liggins 1979).

There is greater unanimity concerning antepartum haemorrhage as a contraindication to β-sympathomimetic treatment. The vasodilator effects of drugs are inappropriate in a patient with haemorrhage, and increased uterine blood flow may increase haemorrhage. The potentially asphyxiating effects of prolonging intra-uterine existence in the presence of antepartum haemorrhage increases the risk of respiratory distress syndrome and neonatal death (Desa 1969).

Using the 1958 perinatal mortality survey statistics (Fedrick and Anderson 1976) we can attempt to estimate the number of patients who might benefit from an effective tocolytic agent. Approximately 1.7 per cent of the study population delivered infants weighing less than 2500 g due primarily to spontaneous preterm labour. Sixty to seventy per cent of patients have ruptured membranes on admission to hospital in preterm labour (O'Driscoll 1977). If even 40 per cent of cases of spontaneous preterm labour are excluded from treatment because of ruptured membranes we are left with only 1 per cent of total births. Almost 30 per cent of spontaneous preterm labours are associated with antepartum haemorrhage, pre-eclamptic toxaemia or maternal diabetes mellitus (Rush et al 1976) which again preclude tocolytic therapy by conventional criteria (Drug and Therapeutics Bulletin 1980). Once patients proved to have a fetus with congenital malformations have been excluded possibly only 4 or 5 patients per 1000 births are eligible for tocolytic therapy. Inevitably, in some of these women labour will be too advanced to permit tocolytic therapy. Thus we have the situation that even a completely effective tocolytic agent would make only a small contribution to the management of preterm labour. Zlatnik (1972) analysed the data from Cornell University in a similar fashion and found that only 12 per cent of total cases of spontaneous preterm labour were likely to show an alteration in outcome if a totally effective tocolytic drug was available.

This has been recognised by those who have made conscientious attempts to assess the efficacy of tocolytic agents. In order to show that a tocolytic agent produces a 25 per cent reduction in perinatal mortality when used for the treatment of preterm labour before 33 weeks maturity a study population of between 80 000 and 110 000 deliveries would be needed (Heyting 1977). Given these requirements it is hardly surprising that a review of controlled clinical trials of drugs used to prevent and to treat preterm labour demonstrated a paucity of convincing evidence of efficacy (Hemminki and Starfield 1978). The statistical requirements of a good controlled trial of a tocolytic agent do not excuse the fact that many studies fail to address themselves to such fundamental issues as perinatal mortality rate, condition of the newborn or proportion of infants weighing more than 2500 g.

A consistent finding of all controlled trials of tocolytic agents (Wesselius de Casparis et al 1971, Fuchs 1976) is the high percentage of 'preterm labour' which is arrested by placebo therapy. This emphasises the difficulty of diagnosing preterm labour accurately. A response to bed rest alone also contributes to the placebo effect.

It invalidates all reports alleging that an agent is an effective tocolytic agent which do not include an appropriate control group. In addition it implies that many women will receive an unnecessary drug and consequently the side effects of tocolytic agents must be viewed in a particularly serious light. The pharmacology, evidence of efficacy and side effects of agents used to suppress preterm labour must be considered in detail.

## PHARMACOLOGICAL AGENTS USED TO INHIBIT UTERINE CONTRACTIONS

### Progestagens

Because progesterone is responsible for the maintenance of electrical and mechanical quiescence of the myometrium in pregnancy, unsuccessful attempts have been made to use this steroid to prevent preterm labour in patients at high risk. Fuchs and Stakeman (1960) attempted to arrest preterm labour with progesterone in oil. There was no consistent response to treatment. The failure of exogenous progesterone to inhibit preterm labour has been ascribed to the impossibility of achieving adequate concentrations of progesterone in the blood in close relation to the myometrium (Hawkins 1974, Darling and Hawkins 1981).

Ovlisen and Iverson (1963) used medroxyprogesterone, also without success. Johnson et al (1975) administered 250 mg of hydroxyprogesterone caproate by weekly injection to 18 patients with a past history of either two spontaneous abortions, two preterm labours, or a combination of these. The treated women had no preterm births while nine of 22 controls delivered preterm infants. Unfortunately, the group treated with progestagen contained more patients with cervical sutures while the control patients had a higher incidence of twin pregnancies and contained more non-Caucasian mothers.

Unwanted effects of drugs are of particular importance when prophylactic use is proposed. Inevitably many women would be exposed to the side effects of progesterone who would never have gone into preterm labour. Large doses of progesterone have a glucocorticoid effect and if they are given orally, antacids should be given to avoid gastric ulceration. An alternative route of administration is rectal. A risk of progestagen therapy is subsequent menstrual irregularity (Turner 1964).

Hydroxyprogesterone and medroxyprogesterone do not cause masculinisation of the female fetus. One hundred and seven infants whose mothers were treated with hydroxyprogesterone in pregnancy have been followed up and found to be normal (Sherman 1966).

**β-sympathomimetics**

Ahlquist's (1948) work on the neurophysiology of the uterus set the scene for the use of β-sympathomimetic agents to suppress uterine activity. The uterus has α-receptors which mediate stimulant effects on the myometrium and β-receptors whose activation inhibits uterine contractions. In the pregnant uterus the situation is more complex. The proportion of β-receptors is changed in pregnancy (Miller and Marshall 1965) and adrenaline itself can activate prostaglandin synthetase and cause release of prostaglandin, with motor effects on the myometrium (Tothill et al 1971). Nonetheless, β-sympathomimetic drugs continue to have an inhibitory effect.

The concept has been introduced of $\beta_1$ receptors subserving the cardiovascular stimulant effects of the drugs and $\beta_2$ receptors mediating inhibitory actions on smooth muscle. This led to the development of relatively specific $\beta_2$ drugs with fewer cardiovascular stimulant properties on the basis of receptor properties. In fact, the evidence that there is any difference between so-called $\beta_1$ and $\beta_2$ receptors is far from clear, and the differential sensitivity to β-sympathomimetics may depend on differences on uptake mechanisms in the tissues.

At least eight β-sympathomimetic agents have been used to suppress uterine activity. They are buphenin, known as nylidrin in the United States of America, feneterol, hexoprenaline, isoxsuprine, orciprenaline, ritodrine, salbutamol and terbutaline. None of these agents lacks cardiovascular and other side effects, although they are more pronounced with the older agents, orciprenaline and isoxsuprine. These less specific drugs cause a greater degree of tachycardia (Gamissans Olivé 1977). In addition to its lack of uterine specificity, isoxsuprine may have the additional effect of having α-sympatholytic activity which contributes to its hypotensive effect, reducing uterine blood flow in some cases (Claassen 1961). A lesser degree of hypotension, mainly diastolic, is seen with the other agents due to peripheral vascular dilatation, but this is partly compensated by the effect on cardiac output, which is increased by as much as 150 per cent with ritodrine (Bieniarz 1977). With this drug the net effect is a widening of the pulse pressure without any change in mean arterial pressure.

The unwanted cardiovascular effects of all these drugs restrict the dose which can be employed to inhibit uterine activity. Figure 12. 1 (from Gamissans Olivé 1978) gives an elegant representation of the ratio between inhibition of uterine activity and increase in maternal pulse rate for four sympathomimetic drugs — terbutaline, ritodrine, orciprenaline and isoprenaline. Of the four drugs, terbutaline has

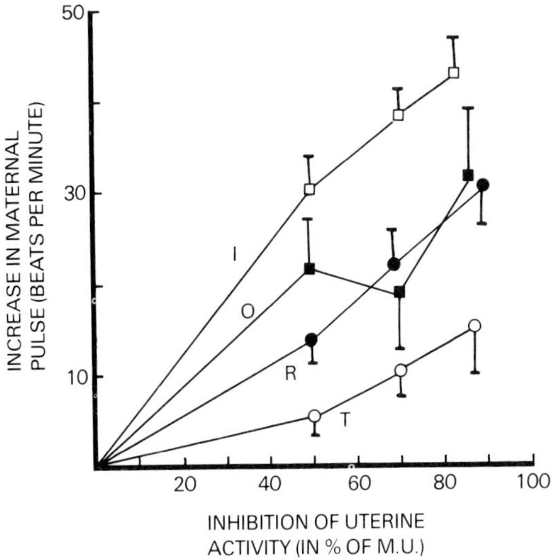


**Fig. 12.1** Increase in maternal pulse and percentage inhibition of uterine activities (in Montevideo units) with isoprenaline (I), orciprenaline (O), ritodrine (R) and terbutaline (T) infused in labour at 2–5 cm cervical diatation in healthy mothers. Terbutaline has the best therapeutic ratio as a uterine relaxant, isoprenaline the worst. (Reproduced with permission from Gamessans Olivé 1978.)

the greatest specificity for uterine inhibition.

Sometimes discomfort, tremor and anxiety in response to the β-sympathomimetic proves to be the dose-limiting factor. It is then worth trying a different drug.

*Pharmacokinetics*

Certain pharmacokinetic properties are shared by all the β-sympathomimetic drugs. Oral preparations of the drugs are absorbed although intravenous administration is usually preferred in the acute situation. As absorption is slower after meals this is the recommended time for oral therapy in order to reduce side effects (Drug and Therapeutics Bulletin 1973) but the dose may need to be increased to achieve therapeutic blood levels.

For all the agents bioavailability is very much greater following a parenteral dose than is the case following oral administration. This effect is due to extensive metabolism of the drug during intestinal absorption or transit through the liver. All the β-sympathomimetic agents are prone to the formation of sulphuric or glucuronic esters. Information about the pharmacokinetics of the drugs in humans is beginning to become available.

*Ritodrine.* When compared with an equivalent parenteral dose, about one third of an oral dose of ritodrine is absorbed and appears in the plasma (Barden et al 1980). Peak plasma levels following oral administration are reached between twenty and eighty minutes and show a two phase decay with half lives at 1.2 hours and 14 hours (Post 1977).

With intramuscular administration peak levels of ritodrine are achieved within five minutes and the half-life is two hours. Intravenously administered ritodrine shows a complex three phase decay with half-lives at 6 to 9 minutes, 1.7 to 2.6 hours and over 3 hours (Barden et al 1980). Irrespective of the route of administration, ritodrine is excreted almost entirely in the urine, either unchanged or as its sulphate or gluconate. Peak excretion is achieved within one hour of administration (Barden et al 1980).

*Salbutamol.* After an oral dose of salbutamol the peak level is reached at one to three hours and the half-life is approximately six hours (Martin et al 1976). Following intravenous administration two half-lives are seen, a brief one at less than an hour and a prolonged half-life at 12 hours (Evans 1973).

*Terbutaline.* Only one twentieth of an oral dose of terbutaline appears in the plasma compared with an equivalent subcutaneous dose. The peak level after oral administration is at 1½ to 2 hours and after subcutaneous administration, 220 minutes. The half-life after oral administration is in excess of 6 hours and after subcutaneous administration is 1½ hours (Leferink 1977).

*Efficacy of the β-sympathomimetics*

*Isoxsuprine* was the first β-sympathomimetic drug used in the treatment of preterm labour (Bishop and Woutersz 1961, Hendricks 1964). Das (1969) found more term deliveries and less perinatal deaths in 24 patients treated with isoxsuprine compared with patients given a variety of analgesics, antispasmodics and sedatives. Csapo and Herczeg (1977) found a significant difference between patients treated with intravenous isoxsuprine compared with controls, in terms of mean birthweight, perinatal mortality, incidence of respiratory distress syndrome — the outcome variables that should be recorded for all trials of tocolytic therapy.

Although in Csapo and Herczeg's (1977) series, maternal side effects were not a serious problem, other authors have found the hypotensive effect of isoxsuprine particularly troublesome (Hendricks 1964). It seems likely that isoxsuprine will be superseded by other more specific agents.

*Orciprenaline* has a slightly more favourable therapeutic ratio than isoxsuprine but has been less rigorously tested as a tocolytic agent.

In an uncontrolled trial 30 patients apparently in labour were treated with orciprenaline. Seventy per cent had labour arrested (Baillie et al 1970). Orciprenaline has usually been given initially in a small test dose of 2.5 $\mu$g/min intravenously with a rapid increase to 80 $\mu$g/min for twenty minutes at a time. This implies a rather different concept of the mode of action of β-sympathomimetics. Most workers with these drugs have used a continuous infusion, steadily increasing the dose until the limit of tolerance, indicated by tachycardia or hypotension, is reached. The infusion rate achieved is usually insufficient to abolish uterine contractions completely, merely reducing their magnitude and frequency, hopefully to an inefficient level. The regimen suggested for orciprenaline is to give a large dose of 20 minutes with the aim of abolishing uterine contractions completely for a short while, even if there are transient side effects. It is hoped in this way to break the cycle of feedback mechanisms (Ferguson 1941) which are reputed to be involved in repetitive uterine contractions, and thus arrest labour permanently.

*Ritodrine* is another $\beta_2$-agonist. The work of Gamissans Olivé (1978) suggests that it shows greater specificity for uterine inhibition than isoprenaline although less specificity than terbutaline (Figure 12. 1). Considerable effort has been expended in subjecting this drug to randomised controlled trials. In 1971, Wesselius de Casparis et al published the results of a multicentre randomised double blind trial conducted in four European countries. Ninety-one women were initially recruited but only 63 remained for the final analysis. Among the patients excluded were patients undergoing caesarean section. Patients who responded to either treatment or placebo and subsequently presented with a new episode of 'preterm labour' were included anew in the analysis and could receive more than one type of treatment. Despite these methodological flaws in the study design this trial must be welcomed as an attempt to assess the value of ritodrine treatment. It is therefore unfortunate that the study did not address itself to important outcome variables such as perinatal mortality and morbidity. Ritodrine arrested preterm labour in 80 per cent of cases while preterm labour was arrested in only 48 per cent of controls given placebo, although the extent of the variation in results between the centres involved is not made clear in its publication.

A larger multicentre trial was conducted in the United States of America (Merkatz et al 1980). Three hundred and thirty six women entered trials in 11 different centres between 1972 and 1979. Patients with twin pregnancies and those with spontaneous rupture of the membranes were subsequently excluded. A variety of treatment protocols were used. In some centres control patients were given a placebo while in others alcohol was given to the controls. Two of the centres studied the effects of oral ritodrine versus placebo in women who had initially been treated with intramuscular ritodrine. In view of the lack of uniformity of the treatment protocols the results must be interpreted with caution. The authors addressed themselves to relevant outcome variables such as neonatal mortality, incidence of respiratory distress syndrome, gestational age at delivery and percentage of infants weighing more than 2500 g. In terms of all these parameters, ritodrine proved superior to treatment with alcohol or placebo. For the relevant outcome variables statistically significant results were achieved only in patients who started treatment before 33 weeks maturity. Some of the individual centres which participated in the study failed to achieve statistically significant results in favour of ritodrine (Lauersen et al 1977, Spellacy et al 1979). This emphasises the very large numbers that are necessary in order to demonstrate a small therapeutic advantage in favour of the use of this or any tocolytic drug in arresting premature labour.

In a recent randomised controlled trial alternative schemes of treatment of preterm labour with ritodrine were compared with bed rest and sedation. None of the ritodrine treatments were demonstrated to be any better than placebo (Larsen et al 1980). The results of this trial are difficult to interpret as the Bishop scores (Bishop 1964) of patients in the ritodrine treated group were apparently higher than those of the controls, suggesting that the cervix was on average more propitious for progress in labour in the test groups before treatment began. Moreover, all cases of congenital malformation and hydramnios occurred in patients treated with ritodrine. This suggests that there might have been some bias in patient allocation. A re-analysis of the results classifying patients according to initial Bishop score showed a statistically significant difference in mean gestational age at delivery in favour of the ritodrine group (Heyting 1980).

*Salbutamol.* McDevitt et al (1975) used salbutamol to suppress uterine contractions in patients in early labour. Uterine activity was not restored by practolol but infusion of propranolol caused an immediate resumption of uterine activity. This was interpreted by the authors as evidence that salbutamol is a selective $\beta_2$-agonist. There is a dearth of randomised controlled trials of salbutamol in arresting premature labour. Liggins and Vaughan (1973) and Korda et al (1974) used intravenous salbutamol and it apparently postponed delivery. Hastwell et al (1978) treated 208 patients with oral salbutamol. Their conclusions with regard to the efficacy of the drug in prolonging pregnancy and reducing the incidence of respiratory distress syndrome are difficult to evaluate without controls. No information is given on the distribution of gestational ages at entry to the trial, although they ranged from 20 to 36 weeks maturity. With 82 per cent of patients delivering at more than 34 weeks it is hardly surprising that the incidence of respiratory distress syndrome in the series was low.

*Terbutaline* appears to be the agent with the most favourable therapeutic ratio (Gamissans Olivé 1978). A small, carefully conducted randomised controlled trial (Ingemarsson, 1976) of 30 patients with some cervical dilatation and effacement, and uterine contractions, between 28 and 36 weeks, showed that pregnancy was prolonged beyond 36 weeks in 12 of the treated group and 3 of the controls. There were higher Apgar scores and birth weights among the treated patients. There no perinatal deaths.

*Other β-sympathomimetic agents* which have been used in the management of preterm labour seem to be broadly similar to ritodrine and terbutaline. Fenoterol is widely used in West Germany (Kubli 1978) but information on its efficacy is scant. In one study comparing buphenin (known as nylidrin in the United States of America) fenoterol and ritodrine, no difference in prolongation of pregnancy was found between the three agents (Richter 1976). In a further study comparing the cardiovascular effects of fenoterol, hexoprenaline, ritodrine and salbutamol, hexoprenaline had the least effect on the maternal cardiovascular system (Lipshitz et al 1976).

*Other therapeutic effects of β-sympathomimetics*

In addition to reducing myometrial contractility two other potentially useful therapeutic effects have been attributed to β-sympathomimetics. These are an increase in uterine blood flow and an acceleration of pulmonary maturation.

*The hypotensive effect* of isoxsuprine causes a reduction in uterine blood flow in a small number of cases (Bishop and Woutersz 1961). Ritodrine may restore uterine blood flow to normal in mild hypertension (Sounio et al 1978). Brettes et al (1976) in a double blind crossover study showed an increase in estimated blood flow during ritodrine infusion in pregnancies complicated by intra-uterine growth retardation. Rats treated with ritodrine during pregnancy showed a slight increase in fetal weight (Barden et al 1980). While feneterol (Lippert et al 1976) and terbutaline (Akerlund and Andersson 1976) may also increase uterine blood flow, salbutamol has been reported to cause a reduction (Elnas et al 1977).

The potential to increase uterine blood flow may have therapeutic applications. Gamissans Olivé et al (1972) demonstrated an improvement in fetal acidosis in labour following administration of ritodrine suggesting improvement in uteroplacental circulation, but Ylikorkala et al (1978) failed to show any alteration in biochemical tests of fetoplacental function after ritodrine or isoxsuprine treatment during pregnancy. Prospective randomised controlled trials will be necessary to evaluate the use of β-sympathomimetics in patients with intra-uterine growth retardation.

*Acceleration of lung maturation.* In 1975 Castren et al reported an increase in the lecithin-sphingomyelin (L/S) ratio in rabbits exposed *in utero* to β-sympathomimetic agents. A small retrospective study by Boog et al (1975) compared 29 preterm infants of ritodrine treated mothers with 34 preterm infants of a control group. There was a statistically significant reduction in respiratory distress syndrome among infants weighing less than 2300 g who were treated with salbutamol, particularly when delivery occurred within 4 hours of the last dose of salbutamol, although the last difference was not statistically significant. Van Iddekinge and Hughes (1977) showed that the infusion of isoxsuprine 40 mg in 1 litre of dextrose at 12 hour intervals for 48 hours was associated with an increase in the lecithin-sphingomyelin ratio in amniotic fluid in eight patients who had an initial L/S ratio of less than 1.4 between 30 and 33 weeks. Six of these women achieved an L/S ratio of more than 2.0 before 34 weeks. Among 45 'control' patients only 3 had an L/S of more than 2.0 before 34 weeks. A larger randomised double-blind trial suggested that orciprenaline had no more effect on the occurrence of respiratory distress syndrome than can be explained by delaying delivery (Schutte et al 198). Larsen et al's (1980) trial showed an increase in respiratory distress syndrome in infants of ritodrine treated mothers but the possible biases in this study have already been discussed.

It is possible that some β-sympathomimetic drugs have an effect on cyclic AMP in the type II pulmonary cells in the fetus and thus accelerate pulmonary maturation. If this is the case, it represents an attractive by-product of tocolytic therapy.

### *Unwanted effects of β-sympathomimetics*

The most important of the unwanted effects of β-sympathomimetics are those on the cardiovascular system. Tachycardia is an unwanted effect shared by all the β-sympathomimetics. Hypotension can occur but may be compensated by an increase in cardiac output with widening of the pulse pressure so that the mean arterial blood pressure is unchanged. The tachycardia associated with therapeutic doses of these agents is distressing. Few patients willingly tolerate a heart rate of more than 150/min. The tachycardia is associated with a change in conduction velocity which can induce arrhythmias, particularly in patients with pre-existing heart disease or in association with hydrocarbon anaesthetic agents (Chez 1978).

Cases of pulmonary oedema have been reported in patients treated with β-sympathomimetics, steroids and intravenous fluids in the management of preterm labour (Elliott et al 1978, Stubblefield 1978, Tinga and Aarnoudse 1979). A further case occurred in a hypertensive woman receiving methyldopa and hydralazine who was treated with salbutamol to inhibit preterm labour (Whitehead et al 1980).

A number of fatalities have been reported in association with β-sympathomimetic treatment. One occurred following delivery in a patient who had been treated with fenoterol and a calcium antagonist. Autopsy revealed a pre-existing cardiomyopathy (Kubli 1978). Cardiomyopathy was also presumed to be a factor in the death of a woman who developed intractable cardiac failure during β-mimetic therapy and died while awaiting heart transplantation (Kubli 1980). At least two other fatalities have occurred (Barden et al 1980) and another near-fatality has been reported (Eskes et al 1980). Although in all cases the cardiomyopathy has been presumed to have existed before the administration of β-sympathomimetics the possibility of a direct toxic effect of the drug on the myocardium in some women has not been excluded.

β-sympathomimetic drugs also have metabolic effects. A highly significant increase in blood glucose, insulin and free fatty acids and a marked decrease in plasma potassium were noted following ritodrine infusion in late pregnancy (Schreyer et al 1979). Lactic acidosis has been reported in a woman treated with ritodrine and corticosteroids (Desir et al 1978). There was no evidence that this woman was diabetic before β-sympathomimetic treatment. Fasting and postprandial blood glucose estimations were normal the day after delivery.

Other unpleasant effects due to sympathetic stimulation are tremor and anxiety with a sense of impending doom in some cases. This is sometimes a dose limiting effect. The unwanted effects of β-sympathomimetic treatment make the contraindications self-evident. Any form of heart disease should ideally be preceded by electrocardiography in all patients. Untreated thyrotoxicosis is a contraindication. Less obviously, perhaps, patients who are already receiving optimal doses of β-sympathomimetic therapy for asthma should not be treated with sympathomimetics to suppress labour as a paradoxical bronchoconstriction can occur.

The metabolic effects of the drugs make their use in patients with diabetes mellitus difficult, but frequent monitoring of blood glucose may permit short term use. Because of the tendency of β-sympathomimetics to cause hypokalaemia, patients on digitalis or diuretics should not be treated without checking plasma potassium levels initially and frequently during treatment.

*Unwanted effects on the fetus*

Unwanted effects on the fetus may be secondary to maternal hypotension or due to the metabolic effects of β-sympathomimetics. Isoxsuprine has a marked hypotensive effect in some patients and unwanted effects on the fetus appear to occur more frequently than with other β-sympathomimetics. A retrospective study has shown an increased risk of hypotension, hypoglycaemia, ileus and neonatal death in infants delivered following isoxsuprine therapy (Brazy and Pupkin 1979) compared with untreated infants of the same maturity. Hypoglycaemia is a common complication, occurring in eight out of twelve babies in one series (Epstein et al 1979). The risk of hypoglycaemia depends on the interval between cessation of β-sympathomimetic therapy and delivery—it was found in five out of six babies delivered within two days of termination of tocolytic therapy and was not present in any of six babies delivered five or more days after ceasing tocolytic therapy (Epstein et al 1979).

Freysz et al (1977) followed up 42 infants of mothers who were treated with β-sympathomimetic drugs. The children, aged from 1 to 3 years, were compared with controls matched for birthweight, sex, gestation at delivery and place of birth. There was no significant difference between the two groups with regard to any of the variables of development studied.

*Conclusions*

Any intending user of β-sympathomimetic drugs should begin by examining both the evidence of their efficacy and their side-effects. The exclusion criteria and the dose schedules already described should be adhered to. If steroids are being used to promote pulmonary maturity, intravenous fluids should be restricted. Intramuscular treatment is pharmacodynamically sound and should be considered as an alternative to intravenous infusion. If oral therapy is employed doses should be given sufficiently frequently to maintain a therapeutic blood level. Electrocardiography is a reasonable precaution before β-sympathomimetic therapy and the plasma potassium should be checked regularly in cases treated for more than 48 hours. As the risk of toxic effects is likely to be related to the duration of therapy, the drug should be discontinued at 34 weeks maturity or sooner if the lecithin-sphingomyelin ratio is mature.

The choice of β-sympathomimetic drug should be based on the evidence of efficacy and the therapeutic ratio. Although ritodrine has been subjected to the most stringent controlled trial (Merkatz et al 1980), terbutaline appears to have a less marked effect on the cardiovascular system (Gamissans Olivé 1978). As this agent has also been the subject of a small well-controlled trial (Ingemarsson 1976) it is not an unreasonable choice of drug for those who wish to use a β-sympathomimetic agent.

**Alcohol**

Ethanol inhibits the release of endogenous oxytocin (Fuchs and Wagner 1963). It also is a smooth muscle relaxant and probably inhibits myometrial contractions directly (Mantell and Liggins 1970). Zlatnik and Fuchs (1972) conducted a randomised controlled trial of intravenous ethanol treatment in patients in preterm labour. Labour was postponed for more than 72 hours in 17 of 21 patients treated with ethanol and in only 8 of 21 patients treated with dextrose and water. Zlatnik and Fuchs (1972) found in their initial study that treatment was ineffective when the membranes were ruptured and in subsequent studies have confined treatment to patients with intact membranes. From 1965 to 1975 they treated a total of 302 patients with 'threatened preterm labour'. In 281 patients with intact membranes 63 per cent had labour postponed for more than 72 hours (Fuchs 1976). There were no controls in this series. Infants weighing over 1000 g at birth had a perinatal mortality rate of 7.3 per cent. Subsequently Fuchs participated in a randomised trial of intravenous ritodrine. Delivery was postponed for more than 72 hours in 77 per cent of the patients given ethanol and 87 per cent of those given ritodrine (Lauersen et al 1977). There was a greater mean gestational age at delivery and a higher mean birth weight in those treated with ritodrine.

Ethanol is administered in an intravenous infusion of a 9.5 per cent solution of ethyl alcohol in 5 per cent dextrose in water with a loading dose of 7.5 ml/kg body weight for 2 hours followed by a maintenance dose of 1.5 ml/kg per hour for 10 hours. If further treatment is required the dose must be reduced. The blood levels at the end of the initial dose were 39 ± 9 mmol/l (178 ± 42 mg/100 ml) and 33 ± 10 mmol/l (150 mg ± 45 mg/100 ml) after the maintenance dose in Fuchs's (1976) series. These levels are well in excess of the legal limits for driving. Given the blood alcohol levels achieved by this regimen it is hardly surprising that the principal side effects of ethanol therapy are inebriation, nausea, restlessness and coma, making this an unpleasant treatment for both patient and nursing staff.

It may be deduced from the randomised controlled trial conducted by Lauersen et al (1977) that the therapeutic ratio of alcohol is unfavourable compared with that of ritodrine. Although there was a statistically significant excess incidence of cardiovascular side-effects in the ritodrine treated patients, in no case did these prevent effective treatment. Ethanol treated patients had a poorer perinatal outcome and a significant increase in nausea, vomiting and urinary incontinence.

Vomiting and aspiration is a potentially lethal complication particularly if delivery by caesarean section becomes necessary. Lactic acidosis occurs in the mother while the baby may exhibit central nervous system depression. While the long-term effects of maternal alcoholism during pregnancy are well documented, the possible long-term effects of a course of intravenous ethanol to suppress labour have not been explored.

### Prostaglandin synthetase inhibitors

As some prostaglandins are potent stimulants of uterine activity and may be involved in the progress of labour, prostaglandin synthetase inhibitors suggest themselves as potential inhibitors of uterine contractions. In animals, aspirin and indomethacin prolong pregnancy and delay labour (Aiken 1972, Novy et al 1974). Zuckerman et al (1974) treated women with suspected pre-term labour with indomethacin. In this uncontrolled trial, uterine contractions were inhibited in forty of the fifty patients. Wiqvist et al (1975) reported a reduction in the amplitude of recorded uterine contractions in six patients treated with indomethacin. Tramontana et al (1979) thought that intravenous infusions of ketoprofen inhibited premature labour in patients with intact membranes. These uncontrolled trials contributed little to the assessment of the value of prostaglandin synthetase inhibitors as tocolytic agents. Niebyl et al (1980) conducted a carefully controlled double-blind randomised trial of indomethacin in patients in preterm labour between 24 and 35 weeks pregnant. The patients had intact fetal membranes with cervical dilatation of more than 2 cm and less than 4 cm. A 24-hour course of indomethacin was more effective than a placebo, with treatment failure occurring in only one of 15 indomethacin-treated patients compared with nine of 15 placebo-treated women. Forty-eight hours after completion of indomethacin therapy the same proportion of patients remained undelivered in the two groups. Ultimately the outcome was the same with respect to gestational age at delivery, birth weight and neonatal morbidity and mortality. This small, meticulously conducted trial took two years to complete at the Johns Hopkins Hospital. It leaves us with no firm evidence that indomethacin is a useful agent for prolonging pregnancy in patients with preterm labour.

The cautious nature of Niebyl et al's (1980) trial can be explained by the widespread concern caused by reports on the possible effects on the fetus of prostaglandin synthetase inhibitors. Several cases of neonatal pulmonary hypertension with a high fatality rate have been reported in infants exposed to salicylates or indomethacin during pregnancy (Arcilla et al 1969, Zuckerman et al 1974, Levin et al 1978). Some of the cases reported were due to chronic salicylate abuse, but one of Levin et al's (1978) fatal cases of neonatal pulmonary hypertension occurred in a patient who received three 25 mg doses of indomethacin to inhibit labour. It is unlikely that this is a chance finding. Prostaglandins are considered to play an important role in regulating tone of the ductus arteriosus *in vivo* (Sharpe and Larsson 1975). Premature closure of the ductus arteriosus *in utero* can provoke lethal neonatal pulmonary hypertension with changes in the pulmonary vascular bed (Levin et al 1978). It seems likely that exposure to prostaglandin synthetase inhibitors can produce premature closure of the ductus arteriosus in some cases.

Careful follow-up examination of the infants in Niebyl et al's (1980) study, with particular emphasis on the cardiopulmonary status, failed to detect any evidence of pulmonary hypertension but as the authors point out, the cardiopulmonary complication rate could be as high as 20 per cent and complications could still have been missed by chance in a study of only 15 infants. Premature closure of the ductus arteriosus is only one of the potential ill-effects on the fetus of prostaglandin synthetase inhibitors. Increase in bleeding time and inhibition of platelet aggregation, impairment of renal function and displacement of bilirubin from its carrier proteins are all possible effects of these drugs. It appears that these effects are more likely to complicate chronic use of the agents throughout pregnancy, than to be associated with acute administration to suppress preterm labour (Wiqvist et al 1978). Obviously, maternal contraindications to some prostaglandin synthetase therapy such as gastrointestinal ulceration continue to apply in pregnancy.

Current evidence on both the efficacy and safety of prostaglandin synthetase inhibitors justify their use only in controlled clinical trials with informed consent from patients. Any further experimental work should probably proceed where Niebyl et al (1980) left off, to see if administration of the drug for more than twenty-four hours will produce a sustained inhibition of uterine activity with an improvement in perinatal outcome. Further evidence on the effects of these agents on the fetus may make even this limited experimental use unethical.

### Magnesium sulphate

Magnesium sulphate is an anticonvulsant with a weak hypotensive effect which makes it a useful adjuvant agent in the treatment of eclampsia. It is thought to inhibit myometrial activity by an effect on acetylcholine release at the neuromuscular junction (Hubbard 1973). In a small randomised trial Steer and Petrie (1977) postponed labour for 24 hours in 24 of 31 patients treated with magnesium sulphate compared with 14 of 31 patients treated with alcohol and 4 of 9 patients treated with intravenous dextrose. No conclusions with regard to efficacy can be drawn without a larger controlled trial which measures appropriate outcome variables in the infant.

Magnesium sulphate may be given by deep intramuscular injection in a dose of 4 to 8 g 8-hourly or by intravenous infusion of a 4 g loading dose followed by a maintenance dose of 1 to 2 g/hour intravenously (Cruikshank et al 1979). The intravenous infusion should be slowed down or stopped if the knee jerks become depressed or if the serum magnesium exceeds 7 mmol/l. Calcium gluconate is the appropriate antidote and 1 g/10 ml of solution should be kept ready at the bedside in case of respiratory depression. Magnesium sulphate crosses the placenta, but the increase in serum magnesium and decrease in serum calcium are both much less than the changes seen in the adult (Cruikshank et al 1979). Neonatal hypomagnesaemia can cause lethargy, flaccidity and diminished respiratory effort. Calcium gluconate may be required. The neonatal dose is 5 to 10 ml of 10 per cent solution given slowly intravenously over 10 minutes. Recently, two cases of pulmonary oedema have been reported in women in preterm labour receiving magnesium sulphate and betamethasone (Elliott et al 1979). In view of the lack of evidence for its efficacy and its potential side-effects there is little to recommend the use of this drug as a tocolytic agent.

### Diazoxide

Diazoxide is a powerful antihypertensive drug which also inhibits uterine activity (Landesman and Wilson 1968). No controlled trials have been carried out to evaluate the use of this drug in preterm labour. Some of the fetal and maternal effects of the drug are already documented because of its use as an antihypertensive agent in severe pre-eclampsia. Chronic administration to sheep and goats causes diabetes in the animals and their offspring. In the human, reversible hyperglycaemia occurs in the mother, with a reactive hypoglycaemia in the infant which may be difficult to treat (Milner and Chouksey 1972, Boulos et at 1971).

**Phosphodiesterase inhibitors**

β-Sympathomimetic-induced myometrial relaxation is associated with an increase in cyclic adenosine monophosphate (AMP) levels in the uterus (Kroeger and Marshall 1974). This raises the possibility of using phosphodiesterase inhibitors such as theophylline and caffeine to inhibit uterine contractions through an increase in uterine cyclic AMP.

Aminophylline (theophylline-ethylenediamine complex) has been given intravenously in a loading dose of 250 mg, either followed by an infusion at a rate of 50 mg hourly or by 250 mg each 6 hours for 48 hours. Treatment may be continued with rectal aminophylline or oral theophylline, 100 mg 8-hourly. The principal side-effect is tachycardia.

Lipshitz (1978) reported on the effect of intravenous aminophylline on oxytocin induced uterine contractions. While a significant reduction in uterine activity was achieved, the therapeutic ratio of this drug was poor compared with an un-named β-sympathomimetic and the author concluded that the unfavourable cardiovascular/tocolytic ratio produced precluded its use in modern obstetric practice.

Sixty-four patients in preterm labour were treated with aminophylline in an uncontrolled trial (Liu and Blackwell, 1978). Approximately 25 per cent of the patients delivered within 24 hours and a further 25 patients were undelivered 7 days after commencing treatment. As there was no control group, it is impossible to say to what extent a placebo effect contributed to the results. No indication of fetal outcome was given. Aminophylline and theophylline cross the placenta (Soyka 1979). This is probably of potential benefit in preterm labour as there is evidence that fetal pulmonary maturation is accelerated by exposure to methylxanthines (Gross and Rooney 1977).

**Calcium antagonists**

Contraction of the myometrium is associated with an influx of calcium ions (Abe 1971). The use of calcium antagonists as tocolytic agents is experimental and at the time of writing is unsupported by any controlled trials.

Verapamil, the calcium antagonist most widely used in the treatment of ischaemic heart disease, seemed to have a potential use as a tocolytic agent but no inhibition of uterine activity was obtained at conventional doses. Higher doses cause impairment of the atrioventricular conduction system. Another calcium antagonist, nifedipine, has less effect on atrioventricular conduction. Andersson (1978) demonstrated a relaxant effect on the uterus *in vitro* and *in vivo* and used nifedipine in 10 women to postpone labour for from 3 to 17 days after the start of treatment. None of the infants delivered following this developed respiratory distress syndrome. Without a controlled trial, this suggested use for calcium antagonists can not be evaluated. Further studies are awaited but it seems likely that the potential cardiovascular effects of these drugs will preclude their use as tocolytic agents.

## CONCLUSIONS

The past decade has seen the emergence of a plethora of drugs which inhibit preterm labour. While β-sympathomimetics, alcohol, and prostaglandin synthetase inhibitors can temporarily inhibit preterm labour, only the β-sympathomimetics have been shown to have a modest benefit on perinatal outcome when compared with placebo therapy. A completely effective β-sympathomimetic agent will alter the outcome in only a very small proportion of total births. The benefit-risk ratio of sympathomimetics is attenuated by the fact that many women will be treated unnecessarily with the agent due to a misdiagnosed or self-limiting episode of preterm labour.

Many obstetricians have been using β-sympathomimetics for years. They are likely to continue so to do now that there is some evidence that perinatal outcome is improved in some cases. Considering the currently documented side-effects of β-sympathomimetic drugs and the potential benefits to be derived from their use it would be equally defensible to withhold them. Improved β-sympathomimetics may emerge, with a greater degree of specificity for the uterus. Even then, only a minority of preterm births will be prevented by tocolysis.

An improvement in general health and living standards may produce a more profound change in the incidence of and mortality from preterm delivery. Improved survival rates will come from better neonatal care and the prevention of trauma and hypoxia in preterm infants.

## REFERENCES

Abe Y 1971 Effects of changing the ionic environment on passive and active membrane properties of pregnant rat uterus. Journal of Physiology 214: 173–190

Ahlquist R P 1948 Study of adrenotropic receptors. American Journal of Physiology 153: 586–600

Aiken J W 1972 Aspirin and indomethacin prolong parturition in rats: evidence that prostaglandins contribute to expulsion of foetus. Nature 240: 21–25

Akerlund M, Andersson K E 1976 Effects of terbutaline on human myometrial activity and endometrial blood flow. Obstetrics and Gynecology 47: 528–535

Anderson A 1978 Epidemiology. Discussion. In: Anderson A, Beard R, Brudenell M, Dunn P (editors) Pre-term labour. Proceedings of the Fifth Study Group of the Royal College of Obstetricians and Gynaecologists. Royal College of Obstetricians and Gynaecologists: London, p. 48

Andersson K E 1978 Inhibition of uterine activity by the calcium antagonist Nifedipine. In: Anderson A, Beard R, Brudenell J and Dunn P (editors) Pre-term labour. Proceedings of the Fifth Study Group of the Royal College of Obstetricians and Gynaecologists. Royal College of Obstetricians and Gynaecologists, London, pp 101–109

Arcilla R A, Thilenius O G, Ranniger K 1969 Congestive heart failure from suspected ductal closure in utero. Journal of Pediatrics 75: 74–78

Baillie P, Meehan F P, Tyack A J 1970 Treatment of premature labour with orciprenaline. British Medical Journal iv: 154–155

Bakketeig, L S, Hoffman H J 1981 Epidemiology of pre-term birth: results from a longitudinal study of births in Norway. In: Elder, M G, Hendricks C H (editors) Pre-term labour. Butterworth, London, pp 17–46

Barden T P, Peter J B, Merkatz J R 1980 Ritodrine hydrochloride: a betamimetic agent for use in pre-term labour. I. Pharmacology, clinical history, administration, side effects and safety. Obstetrics and Gynecology 56: 1–6

Bender S 1952 Twin pregnancy. Journal of Obstetrics and Gynaecology of the British Empire 59: 510–517

Bieniarz J 1977 Cardiovascular effects of beta-adrenergic agonists. In: Anderson A, Beard R, Brudenell J, Dunn P (editors) Pre-term labour. Proceedings of the Fifth Study Group of the Royal College of Obstetricians and Gynaecologists. Royal College of Obstetricians and Gynaecologists, London, pp 188–202

Bishop E H 1964 Pelvic scoring for elective induction. Obstetrics and Gynecology 24: 266–268

Bishop E H, Woutersz T B 1961 Isoxsuprine, a myometrial relaxant. Obstetrics and Gynecology 17: 442–446

Boog G, Ben Brahim M, Gandar R 1975 Beta-mimetic drugs and possible prevention of respiratory distress syndrome. British Journal of Obstetrics and Gynaecology 82: 285–288

Boulos B M, Davis L E, Almond C H, Jackson R L 1971 Placental transfer of diazoxide and its hazardous effects on the newborn. Journal of Clinical Pharmacology 11: 206–210

Brazy J E, Pupkin M J 1979 Effects of maternal isoxsuprine administration on pre-term infants. Journal of Pediatrics 94: 444–449

Brettes J P, Renaud R, Gordon R 1976 A double blind investigation into the effects of ritodrine on uterine blood flow during the third trimester of pregnancy. American Journal of Obstetrics and Gynecology 124: 164–168

British Medical Journal 1979 Premature rupture of the membranes (editorial). British Medical Journal i: 1165–1166

Browne E J, Dixon H G 1963 Twin pregnancy. Journal of Obstetrics and Gynaecology of the British Commonwealth 70: 251–257

Brumfitt W, Reeves D S 1968 Screening procedures for urinary infection. In: Sharp

E L, Keen H (editors) Presymptomatic and early diagnosis. A critical appraisal. Pitman, London, pp 179–201
Castren O, Gummerus M, Saarikoski S 1975 Treatment of imminent premature labour. Acta Obstetricia et Gynecologica Scandinavica 54: 95–100
Chamberlain G 1979 Background to perinatal health. Lancet ii: 1061–1063
Chamberlain G, Philipp E, Howlett B, Masters K 1978 British births 1970. Volume II: Obstetric care. Heinemann Medical, London, p. 261
Chez R 1978 The effect of beta-sympathomimetic drugs on carbohydrate metabolism in pregnancy. Discussion. In: Anderson A, Beard R, Brudenell J, Dunn P (editors) Pre-term labour. Proceedings of the Fifth Study Group of the Royal College of Obstetricians and Gynaecologists. Royal College of Obstetricians and Gynaecologists, London, pp 212–215
Claassen V 1961 Stero-specific devergence in the actions of adrenergic alpha and beta receptors. Biochemical Pharmacology 8: 116
Creasy R K, Liggins G C 1979 Aetiology and management of preterm labour. In: Stallworthy J, Bourne G (editors) Recent advances in obstetrics and gynaecology. Churchill Livingstone, Edinburgh, pp 21–45
Cruikshank D P, Pitkin R M, Reynolds W A, Williams G A, Hargis G K 1979 Effects of magnesium sulfate treatment on perinatal calcium metabolism. I. Maternal and fetal responses. American Journal of Obstetrics and Gynecology 134: 243–249
Csapo A I, Herczeg J 1977 Arrest of premature labour by isoxsuprine. American Journal of Obstetrics and Gynecology 129: 482–491
Darling M R, Hawkins D F 1981 Sex hormones in pregnancy. Clinics in Obstetrics and Gynaecology. Saunders, London
Das R K 1969 Isoxsuprine in premature labour. Journal of Obstetrics and Gynaecology of India 19: 566–570
Desa, D J 1969 An analysis of certain factors in the aetiology of respiratory distress syndrome of the newborn. Journal of Obstetrics and Gynaecology of the British Commonwealth 76: 148
Desir D, Van Coevorden A, Kirkpatrick C, Caufriez A 1978 Ritodrine induced acidosis in pregnancy. British Medical Journal ii: 1194–1195
Donovan J W 1977 Randomized controlled trial of anti-smoking advice in pregnancy. British Journal of Preventive and Social Medicine 31: 6–12
Drillien C M 1972 Aetiology and outcome in low birthweight infants. Developmental Medicine and Child Neurology 14: 563–574
Drug and Therapeutics Bulletin 1973 Arresting premature labour. Orciprenaline and other drugs. Drug and Therapeutics Bulletin 11: 25–26
Drug and Therapeutics Bulletin 1980 The arrest of preterm labour. Drug and Therapeutics Bulletin 18: 34–36
Dumont M, Poizet C L 1974 Etude d'un coefficient d'appréciation de la béance cervico-isthmique. Journal de Gynécologie, Obstétrique et Biologie de la Réproduction 3: 981–995
Eggers T R, Doyle L W, Pepperell R J 1979 Premature rupture of the membranes. Medical Journal of Australia i: 209–312
Elliott H R, Abdullah U, Hayes P J 1978 Pulmonary oedema associated with ritodrine infusion and betamethasone administration in premature labour. British Medical Journal ii: 799–800
Elliott J P, O'Keefe D F, Greenberg P, Freeman R K 1979 Pulmonary edema associated with magnesium sulfate and betamethasone treatment. American Journal of Obstetrics and Gynecology 134: 717–718
Elnas S, Joelsson L, Lewander K, Lundqist H, Lunell N, Sarby B, Astrom H 1977 The effect of beta-receptor stimulating agents on the uteroplacental blood flow. Acta Obstetricia et Gynecologica Scandinavica 56: 297–301.
Epstein M F, Nicholls E, Stubblefield P G 1979 Neonatal hypoglycaemia after beta-sympathomimetic tocolytic therapy. Journal of Pediatrics 94: 449–453
Eskes T K, Kornman J J, Bots K S, Hein P R, Gimbrere J S, Vork J T 1980

Maternal morbidity due to beta-adrenergic therapy. Pre-existing cardiomyopathy aggravated by fenoterol. European Journal of Obstetrics, Gynecology and Reproductive Biology 10: 41–46
Evans M E 1973 The metabolism of salbutamol in man. Xenobiotica 3: 113–120
Fedrick J 1976 Antenatal identification of women at high risk of spontaneous preterm birth. British Journal of Obstetrics and Gynaecology 83: 351–354
Fedrick J, Anderson A 1976 Factors associated with spontaneous pre-term births. British Journal of Obstetrics and Gynaecology 83: 342–350
Ferguson J K W 1941 A study of the motility of the intact uterus at term. Surgery, Gynecology and Obstetrics 73: 359–363
Freysz H, Willard D, Lehr A, Messer J, Boog G 1977 A long term evaluation of infants who received a beta-mimetic while in utero. Journal of Perinatal Medicine 5: 94–99
Fuchs A-R, Wagner G 1963 Effects of alcohol on release of oxytocin. Nature 198: 92–93
Fuchs F 1976 Prevention of prematurity. American Journal of Obstetrics and Gynecology 126: 809–820
Fuchs F, Stakeman G 1960 Treatment of threatened premature labour with large doses of progresterone. American Journal of Obstetrics and Gynecology 79: 172–176
Furness E T, McDonald P J, Beasley N V 1975 Urinary antiseptics in asymptomatic bacteruria in pregnancy. New Zealand Medical Journal 81: 417–419
Gamissans Olivé O 1978 Beta-adrenergic agonists. Discussion. In: Anderson A, Beard R, Brudenell J, Dunn P (editors) Pre-term labour. Proceedings of the Fifth Study Group of the Royal College of Obstetricians and Gynaecologists. Royal College of Obstetricians and Gynaecologists, London, pp 171–182
Gamissans Olivé O, Carreras M, Duran P, Cararach J, Calaf J, Abril V, Esteban-Altirriba J 1972 The treatment of fetal acidosis with beta-mimetic drugs. Studies on acid-base balance, blood glucose levels and uterine motility. In: Baumgarten K, Wesselius de Casparis A (editors) Proceedings of the International Symposium on the Treatment of Fetal Risks. University of Vienna, pp 145–148
Gamsu H R, Light F, Fotter A, Price J F 1979 Intensive care and the very low birthweight infant. Lancet ii: 736
Gold E M, Traub F B, Daichman I, Terris M 1966 Asymptomatic bacteriuria during pregnancy. Obstetrics and Gynecology 27: 206–209
Goodlin R C, Keller D W, Raffin M 1971 Orgasm during late pregnancy: possible deleterious effects. Obstetrics and Gynecology 38: 916–920
Gross I, Rooney S 1977 Aminophylline stimulates phospholipid synthesis by fetal rat lung in organ culture. Pediatric Research 11: 571
Hansard 1978 Written answers, column 233, 13 December. Her Majesty's Stationary Office, London
Hastwell G B, Holloway C P, Taylor T L O 1978 A study of 208 patients in premature labour treated with orally administered salbutamol. Medical Journal of Australia i: 465–469
Hawkins D F 1974 Sex hormones in pregnancy. In: D F Hawkins (editor) Obstetric therapeutics. Baillière Tindall, London, p. 128
Hemminki E, Starfield B 1978 Prevention and treatment of premature labour by drugs: review of controlled clinical trials. British Journal of Obstetrics and Gynaecology 85: 411–417
Hendricks C H 1964 The use of isoxsuprine for the arrest of premature labour. Clinical Obstetrics and Gynecology 7: 687–694
Heyting A 1980 Ritodrine in preterm labour. A clinical trial to compare a standard treatment with three regimens involving the use of ritodrine. British Journal of Obstetrics and Gynaecology 87: 1056
Heyting M 1977 The problems of a prospective study in perinatal mortality. In: Bompiani A, Cosmi E, Fischetti B, Gasperi F, Romerini C (editors) Recent

advances on beta-mimetic drugs in obstetrics. Societá Editrie Universe, Rome, p. 173.
House of Commons 1980 Second report from the Social Services Committee. Session 1979–1980. Perinatal and Neonatal Mortality ('Short Report') Her Majesty's Stationery Office, London, volume I, p. 115
Hubbard J I 1973 Microphysiology of vertebrate neuromuscular transmission. Physiological Reviews 53: 674–723
Illsley R, Thompson B 1976 Social characteristics identifying women at risk of premature delivery. In: Turnbull A C, Woodward F P (editors) Prevention of handicap through antenatal care. Associated Scientific Publishers, Amsterdam, pp 149–155
Ingemarsson I 1976 Effect of terbutaline on premature labour. American Journal of Obstetrics and Gynecology 125: 520–524
Jeffrey R L, Bowes W A I, Delaney J J 1973 Role of bed rest in twin gestation. Obstetrics and Gynecology 43: 822–826
Johnson J W C, Austin K L, Jones G S 1975 Efficacy of 17α-hydroxy-progesterone caproate in the prevention of premature labor. New England Journal of Medicine 293: 675–680
Jones R A, Cummins M, Davies P 1979 Infants of very low birthweight. Lancet i: 1332–1335
Kaltreider D F, Kohl S 1980 Epidemiology of preterm delivery. Clinical Obstetrics and Gynecology 23: 17–31
Kaminski M, Papiernik E 1974 Multifactorial study of risk of prematurity at 32 weeks. I. Journal of Perinatal Medicine 2: 37–44
Kaminski M, Goujard J, Rumeau-Rouquette C 1973 Prediction of low birthweight and prematurity by a multiple regression analysis with maternal characteristics known since the beginning of pregnancy. International Journal of Epidemiology 2: 195–204
Kass E H 1960 Bacteruria and pyelonephritis of pregnancy. Archives of Internal Medicine 105: 42–46
Kass E H 1973 The role of unsuspected infection in the etiology of prematurity. Clinical Obstetrics and Gynecology 16: 134–152
Komaŕomy B, Lampé L 1977 The value of rest in twin pregnancies. International Journal of Gynaecology and Obstetrics 15: 262–266
Korda A R, Lynehan R C, Jones W R 1974 The treatment of premature labour with intravenously administered salbutamol. Medical Journal of Australia i: 744–747
Kroeger E A, Marshall J M 1974 Beta-adrenergic effects on rat myometrium: role of c AMP. American Journal of Physiology 226: 1298–1303
Kubli F 1978 The effect of beta-sympathomimetic drugs on carbohydrate metabolism in pregnancy. Discussion. In: Anderson A, Beard R, Brudenell J, Dunn P (editors) Pre-term labour. Proceedings of the Fifth Study Group of the Royal College of Obstetricians and Gynaecologists. Royal College of Obstetricians and Gynaecologists, London, p. 218
Kubli F 1980 Maternal morbidity due to beta-adrenergic therapy. Pre-existing cardiomyopathy aggravated by fenoterol. Commentary. European Journal of Obstetrics, Gynaecology and Reproductive Biology 10: 44–45
Landesman R, Wilson K H 1968 The relaxant effect of diazoxide on isolated gravid and non-gravid human myometrium. American Journal of Obstetrics and Gynecology 101: 120–125
Larsen J F, Hansen M K, Hesseldahl H, Kristoffersen K, Larsen P K, Osler M, Weber J, Eldsa K, Large A 1980 Ritodrine in the treatment of preterm labour. A clinical trial to compare a standard treatment with three regimens involving the use of ritodrine. British Journal of Obstetrics and Gynaecology 87: 949–957
Lauersen N, Merkatz I, Tejani N, Wilson K, Roberson A, Mann L, Fuchs F 1977 Inhibition of premature labour. A multicentre comparison of ritodrine and ethanol. American Journal of Obstetrics and Gynecology 127: 837–834

Laursen B 1973 Twin pregnancy. The value of prophylactic rest in bed and the risk involved. Acta obstetricia et gynecologica Scandinavica 52: 367–371
Law R G 1967 Standards of obstetric care. The report of the North West Metropolitan Regional Hospital Survey 1962–1964. Livingstone, Edinburgh, Part I, section 60, p. 188
Leferink J G 1977 Quantitative analysis of terbutaline in serum and urine at therapeutic levels using gas chromatography-mass spectrometry. Journal of Chromatography 143: 299–305
Levin D L, Fixler D E, Moriss F C, Tyson J 1978 Morphologic analysis of the pulmonary vascular bed in infants exposed in utero to prostaglandin synthetase inhibitors. Journal of Pediatrics 22: 478–483
Lewis P, De Swiet M, Boylan P, Bulpitt C J 1980 How obstetricians in the United Kingdom manage preterm labour. British Journal of Obstetrics and Gynaecology 87: 574–577
Liggins G C, Vaughan G S 1973 Intravenous infusion of salbutamol in the management of premature labour. Journal of Obstetrics and Gynaecology of the British Commonwealth 80: 29–32
Lippert T H, de Grandi P B, Fridrich R 1976 Actions of the uterine relaxant fenoterol on uteroplacental dynamics in human subjects. American Journal of Obstetrics and Gynecology 125: 1093–1098
Lipshitz J 1978 Uterine and cardiovascular effects of aminophylline. American Journal of Obstetrics and Gynecology 131: 716–718
Lipshitz J, Baillie P, Davey D A 1976 A comparison of uterine $beta_2$ adrenoreceptor selectivity of fenoterol, hexoprenaline, ritodrine and salbutamol. South African Journal of Obstetrics and Gynecology, supplement 65 50: 1969–1972
Liu D T, Blackwell R J 1978 The value of a scoring system in predicting outcome of pre-term labour and comparing efficacy of treatment with aminophylline and salbutamol. British Journal of Obstetrics and Gynaecology 85: 418–414
McDevitt D G, Wallace R I, Roberts A, Whitfield C R 1975 The uterine and cardiovascular effect of salbutamol and practolol during labour. British Journal of Obstetrics and Gynaecology 82: 442–448
Mantell C D, Liggins G C 1970 The effect of ethanol on the myometrial response to oxytocin in women at term. Journal of Obstetrics and Gynaecology of the British Commonwealth 77: 976–981
Martin L E, Rees J, Tanner R J 1976 Quantitative determination of salbutamol in plasma as either trimethylsilyl or t-butyldimethylsilyl ether, using a stable isotope multiple ion recording technique. Biomedical Mass Spectrometry 3: 184–190
Merkatz I R, Peter J B, Barden T P 1980 Ritodrine hydrochloride: a betamimetic agent for use in preterm labor. II Evidence of efficacy. Obstetrics and Gynecology 56: 7–12
Miller M D, Marshall J M 1965 Uterine response to nerve stimulation: relation to hormonal status and catecholamines. American Journal of Physiology 209: 859
Milner R D G, Chouksey S K 1972 Effects of fetal exposure to diazoxide in man. Archives of Disease in Childhood 47: 537–543
Naeye R L 1979 Coitus and associated amniotic fluid infection. New England Journal of Medicine 301: 1198–1200
Newcombe R, Chalmers I 1981 Assessing risk of pre-term labour. In: Elder M G, Hendricks C H (editors) Pre-term labour. Butterworth, London, pp 47–60
Newton R W, Webster P A, Binn P S, Maskrey N, Phillips A B 1979 Psychosocial stress in pregnancy and its relation to the onset of premature labour. British Medical Journal ii: 412–413
Niebyl J R, Blake D A, White R D, Kumor K M, Dubin N H, Robinson J C, Egner P G 1980 The inhibition of premature labor with indomethacin. American Journal of Obstetrics and Gynecology 136: 1014–1019
Novy M J, Cook M J, Manugh L 1974 Indomethacin block of normal parturition in primates. American Journal of Obstetrics and Gynecology 118: 412–416
O'Driscoll K M 1977 Physiology and pharmacology. Discussion. In: Anderson A,

Beard R, Brudenell J, Dunn P (editors) Pre-term labour. Proceedings of the Fifth Study Group of the Royal College of Obstetricians and Gynaecologists. Royal College of Obstetricians and Gynaecologists, London, p. 126

Ovlisen B, Iverson J 1963 Treatment of threatened premature labour with 6αmethyl-17α-acetoxyprogesterone. American Journal of Obstetrics and Gynecology 86: 291–295

Papiernik E 1977 Epidemiology. Discussion. In: Anderson A, Beard R, Brudenell J, Dunn P (editors) Pre-term labour. Proceedings of the Fifth Study Group of the Royal College of Obstetricians and Gynaecologists. Royal College of Obstetricians and Gynaecologists, London, p. 148

Post L C 1977 Pharmacokinetics of beta-adrenergic agonists. In: Anderson A, Beard R, Brudenell J, Dunn P (editors) Pre-term Labour. Proceedings of the Fifth Study Group of the Royal College of Obstetricians and Gynaecologists. Royal College of Obstetricians and Gynaecologists, London, pp 134–147

Renaud R, Irrman M, Gander K, Flynn M G 1974 The use of ritodrine in the treatment of premature labour. Journal of Obstetrics and Gynaecology of the British Commonwealth 81: 182–186

Reynolds O, Stewart A 1980 Comparison of neonatal management methods for very low birth weight babies. British Medical Journal ii: 1488–1489

Richter R 1976 Evaluation of success in treatment of threatening premature labor by betamimetic drugs. American Journal of Obstetrics and Gynecology 127: 482–486

Ritchie K, McClure G 1979 Prematurity. Lancet ii: 1227–1229

Robertson J G, Livingstone J R B, Isdale M H 1968 The management and complications of asymptomatic bacteruria in pregnancy. Journal of Obstetrics and Gynaecology of the British Commonwealth 75: 59–65

Rush D, Stein Z, Susser M 1980 A randomised controlled trial of prenatal nutritional supplementation in New York City. Pediatrics 65: 683–697

Rush R W, Keirse M J, Howat P, Baum J D, Anderson A, Turnbull A C 1976 Contribution of preterm delivery to perinatal mortality. British Medical Journal ii: 965–968

Schreyer P, Caspi E, Ariely S, Herzianu I, User P, Gilboa Y, Zaidman J L 1979 Metabolic effects of intravenous ritodrine infusion during pregnancy. European Journal of Obstetrics, Gynecology and Reproductive Biology 9: 97–103

Schutte M F, Treffers P E, Koppe J G, Bruer W 1980 The influence of betamethasone and orciprenaline on the incidence of respiratory distress syndrome in the newborn after preterm labour. British Journal of Obstetrics and Gynaecology 130: 745–747

Sharpe G L, Larsson K S 1975 Studies on closure of the ductus arteriosus. X. In vivo effect of prostaglandin. Prostaglandins 9: 703–719

Sherman A J 1966 Hormonal therapy for control of incompetent os of pregnancy. Obstetrics and Gynecology 28: 198–205

Sounio O, Olkkonen H, Lahtinen T 1978 Maternal circulatory response to a single dose of ritodrine hydrochloride during orthostasis in normal and hypertensive late pregnancy. American Journal of Obstetrics and Gynecology 130: 745–747

Soyka L F 1979 Effects of methylxanthines on the fetus. Clinics in Perinatology 6: 37–51

Spellacy W N, Cruz A C, Birk S A, Buhl W C 1979 Treatment of premature labor with ritodrine. A randomised controlled study. Obstetrics and Gynaecology 54: 220–223

Steer C M, Petrie R H 1977 A comparison of magnesium sulphate and alcohol for the prevention of premature labour. American Journal of Obstetrics and Gynaecology 129: 1–4

Stewart A L, Turcan D M, Rawlings G, Reynolds E O R 1977 Prognosis for infants weighing 100 g or less at birth. Archives of Disease of Childhood 52: 97–104

Stubblefield P G 1978 Pulmonary edema occurring after therapy with

dexamethasone and terbutaline for premature labor. A case report. American Journal of Obstetrics and Gynecology 132: 341–342
Tinga D J, Aarnoudse J G 1979 Post-partum pulmonary oedema associated with preventive therapy for premature labour. Lancet i: 1026
Tothill A, Rathbone L, Willman, Eve 1971 Relation between prostaglandin $E_2$ and adrenaline reversal in the rat uterus. Nature 233: 56–57
Tramontana S, Allocca G, Caserta R, Borelli A L, Raucci F 1979 L'uso del ketoprofene nella minaccia di parto pretermine. Minerva Ginecologia 31: 291
Turnbull A 1977 Epidemiology. Discussion. In: Anderson A, Beard R, Brudenell J, Dunn P (editors) Pre-term labour. Proceedings of the Fifth Study Group of the Royal College of Obstetricians and Gynaecologists. Royal College of Obstetricians and Gynaecologists, London, p. 48
Turner S J 1964 Prolonged postpartum dysfunctional uterine bleeding subsequent to prenatal therapy with parenteral potent progestogens. Obstetrics and Gynecology 24: 218–221
Van Iddekinge B, Hughes E A 1977 The effect of intrauterine fetal transfusion and a beta-sympathomimetic substance on the lecithin sphingomyelin ratio in human amniotic fluid. British Journal of Obstetrics and Gynaecology 84: 669–673
Weekes A R L, Menzies D N, De Boer C H 1977 The selective efficacy of bed-rest, cervical suture and no treatment in the management of twin pregnancy. British Journal of Obstetrics and Gynaecology 84: 161–164
Wesselius de Casparis A, Thiery M, Yo Le Sian A, Baumgarten K, Brosens I, Gammissans O, Stalk J G, Vivian W 1971 Results of a double-blind multi-centre study with ritodrine in premature labour. British Medical Journal iii: 144–147
Whitehead M, Mander A M, Hertogs K, Williams R M, Pettingale K W 1980 Lesson of the week. Acute congestive cardiac failure in a hypertensive woman receiving salbutamol for premature labour. British Medical Journal i: 1221–1222
Wiqvist N 1978 Effects of prostaglandins and synthetase inhibitors on the fetal circulation. Discussion. In: Anderson A, Beard R, Brudenell J, Dunn P (editors) Pre-term labour. Proceedings of the Fifth Study Group of the Royal College of Obstetricians and Gynaecologists. Royal College of Obstetricians and Gynaecologists, London, p. 243
Wiqvist N, Lundstrom V, Green K 1975 Premature labour and indomethacin. Prostaglandins 10: 515–526
Ylikorkala O, Kauppila A, Tuimala R, Haapalathi J, Karppanen H, Viinikka L 1978 Effects of intravenous isoxsuprine and ritodrine on placental and pituitary hormones and cyclic adenosine monophosphate. American Journal of Obstetrics and Gynecology 130: 302–306
Zlatnik F J 1972 The applicability of labour inhibition to the problem of prematurity. American Journal of Obstetrics and Gynecology 113: 704–706
Zlatnik F J, Fuchs F 1972 A controlled trial of ethanol in threatened premature labor. American Journal of Obstetrics and Gynecology 112: 610–612
Zuckerman H, Reiss U, Rubinstein I 1974 Inhibition of human premature labour by indomethacin. Obstetrics and Gynecology 44: 787–792

# 13

*R. F. Lamont*

# Drugs in pregnancy and neonatal jaundice

## BILIRUBIN METABOLISM

### Bilirubin metabolism in the fetus

Bilirubin found in the reticulo-endothelial system of the fetus from breakdown of haem-containing compounds is transported in early fetal life, bound to α-fetoprotein, to sites of excretion. Later in fetal life, as α-fetoprotein concentration falls and albumin concentration rises, albumin binding takes over the main role of transportation of bilirubin (Schenker et al 1964).

Bilirubin within the circulation of the fetus can be disposed of by either of two routes. The placenta is freely permeable to unconjugated bilirubin when dissociated from albumin. The higher concentration of maternal serum albumin (40 g/l) compared to that of the fetus (30 g/l) favours clearance by and transport of fetal bilirubin away from the placenta for detoxification and excretion by the maternal liver. The other route for clearance of fetal bilirubin is by the fetal liver, but this mechanism is less efficient than in the neonate or in adults. Circulation through venous sinusoids of the fetal liver and therefore access to liver cells (hepatocytes) in the liver parenchyma is reduced because the bulk of the portal circulation, supplying 80 per cent of hepatic blood flow, is being shunted through the ductus venosus. Also, the supply of blood from the fetal hepatic artery, chiefly to the right lobe, enters the sinusoidal circulation distally, further reducing effective perfusion of the liver parenchyma. Another impediment to abundant sinusoidal perfusion and exchange of bilirubin in the fetal liver is the mechanical effect of large amounts of extramedullary haemopoietic tissue in the sinusoids.

After fifteen weeks of pregnancy the fetal liver glucuronidates bilirubin and excretes it in bile (Felsher et al 1978). This passage of bilirubin into bile necessitates an enterohepatic circulation of bilirubin, since without such a circulation a continuous pigmented gallstone would develop in the fetal intestine.

Since no anaerobic bacteria exist in the fetal intestine to reduce conjugated bilirubin to urobilinogen, urobilins and stercobilins, the enzyme required must be derived from elsewhere; a β-glucuronidase which can subserve this function has been shown to exist in meconium (Takimoto and Matsuda 1971).

The unconjugated bilirubin yielded by this enzymatic cleavage in the fetal intestine is reabsorbed into the fetal circulation and must again be cleared by the placenta or fetal liver. Some of the urobilinogen is absorbed and is either excreted by the fetal liver into bile or by the fetal kidney into urine. Thus the fetus is limited in its routes for excreting bilirubin to the passage of albumin-free, unconjugated bilirubin through the placenta, and to renal excretion of a small amount of urobilinogen into the amniotic fluid.

### Bilirubin metabolism in the neonate

After delivery the neonate must rely fully on its own liver for detoxification and excretion of bilirubin. In the neonate 75 per cent of bilirubin is formed from the breakdown of fetal haemoglobin (Brown 1962). The normal term infant breaks down about 0.5 g of haemoglobin each day, yielding about 16 mg of bilirubin. The remaining 25 per cent of bilirubin is derived from other compounds containing haem such as myoglobin and cytochromes. One molecule of albumin binds two molecules of bilirubin; one of these molecules is 300 times more tightly bound than the other (Jacobsen 1969). The latter molecule can easily be displaced by competitors for the same binding site like free fatty acids and some drugs, most notably sulphonamides.

In the newborn, unconjugated albumin-bound bilirubin is delivered to the cell membrane of the hepatocytes in the liver parenchyma where it is detached from albumin, bound to the cytoplasmic proteins ligandin (Y-protein) and Z-protein and transported to the microsomes of the cell cytoplasm to undergo detoxification (Levi et al 1969). Next the bilirubin is conjugated with one or two molecules of glucuronic acid by the enzyme bilirubin-uridine-diphosphate-glucuronyl transferase and excreted in bile via the biliary tree into the intestine.

In the neonatal intestine, bacterial β-glucuronidase deconjugates most of the bilirubin to urobilinogen, which is absorbed into the blood, and passes in the portal circulation to the liver for excretion in bile and to the systematic circulation for excretion in urine.

## NEONATAL JAUNDICE

### Physiological jaundice in the neonate

Disturbance of these physiological mechanisms may cause jaundice, and can be divided into one or more of three main aetiologies (Table

**Table 13.1** Causes of neonatal jaundice

| | |
|---|---|
| *Prehepatic* | Increased bilirubin production |
| *Hepatic* | (a) Disturbance of transport of bilirubin into the microsomes of the liver cells |
| | (b) Disturbance of enzymatic conjugation |
| *Posthepatic* | Reduced excretion of conjugated bilirubin in bile into the intestine |

13.1. The commonest cause of neonatal jaundice is 'physiological jaundice.' This occurs for a number of reasons:

(1) Increased haemoglobin concentration, for example from delayed clamping of the cord; the incidence of jaundice is six times greater if the cord is clamped more than one minute after delivery.
(2) Shortened red cell half-life—45 to 70 days in the neonate compared to 120 days in the adult (Bratteby et al 1968).
(3) Concealed haemorrhage in the newborn—even normal deliveries are associated with extravasation of red cells into the tissues.
(4) Low levels of ligandin and glucuronyl transferase in the liver of the newborn in the first week of life (Odell et al 1976).
(5) Breast milk jaundice—probably due to the lipid component of milk inhibiting glucuronyl transferase activity (Luzeau et al 1974) occurring in some women.

In the preterm infant some of these factors are accentuated. The haemoglobin concentration is often greater, and the red cell half life is only 30 to 40 days. Conjugation of bilirubin is less efficient than in term infants and this is also true of other exogenous and endogenous compounds which normally undergo glucuronidation. The proportion of conjugated to unconjugated bilirubin is less in bile, and there are increased levels of bilirubin diglucuronide over monoglucuronide, probably representing immature conjugation mechanisms.

The most important mechanism of jaundice in preterm occurs because the shorter the gestation, the lower are babies liver uridine-diphosphate-glucuronyl-transferase levels. Even in term babies, adult levels of this enzyme are not reached until the tenth week of extra-uterine life, long after the usual time of disappearance of 'physiological jaundice' (Stern et al 1970). Hepatic immaturity may also be due to diminished perfusion of and uptake by the liver cell, a process which can be stimulated by drugs such as phenobarbitone.

**Table 13.2** Pathological causes of neonatal jaundice

I *Prehepatic*
- A. Haemolysis
    1. Feto-maternal blood group incompatibility: Rhesus, ABO, minor blood groups
    2. Hereditory spherocytosis
    3. Red cell enzyme deficiencies: glucose-6-phosphate dehydrogenase deficiency
    4. Abnormal haemoglobins: thalassaemia
- B. Polycythaemia
    1. Delayed cord clamping
    2. Materno-fetal transfusion
    3. Feto-fetal transfusion in multiple pregnancy
- C. Haematomata

II *Hepatic*
- A. Inborn errors
    1. Familial non-haemolytic jaundice; Crigler-Najjar syndrome, autosomal dominant type Dubin-Johnson syndrome
    2. Galactosaemia
    3. Tyrosinaemia
    4. Hereditary fructose intolerance
- B. Metabolic and hormonal
    1. Hypothyroidism
    2. Hypopituitarism
    3. Breast milk jaundice
    4. Infants of diabetic mothers
    5. $\alpha_1$-antitrypsin deficiency

III *Posthepatic*
- A. Biliary atresia
- B. Cholangitis
- C. Choledochal cyst
- D. Cystic fibrosis
- E. Tumour
- F. Cholestasis

IV *Mixed*
- A. Drugs given to mother
- B. Drugs given to neonate
- C. Jaundice of prematurity
- D. Sepsis
    1. Acquired or congenital
    2. Viral, bacterial, fungal or protozoal
- E. Congenital hepatitis or cirrhosis
- F. Right heart failure
- G. Increased enterohepatic circulation of bilirubin
    1. Swallowed blood
    2. Pyloric stenosis
    3. Intestinal atresia or stenosis
    4. Cystic fibrosis: meconium ileus, meconium plug syndrome
    5. Hirschprung's disease
    6. Annular pancreas
    7. Paralytic ileus

**Differential diagnosis of neonatal jaundice**

Pathological causes of neonatal jaundice (Table 13.2) may co-exist with physiological jaundice. The conditions associated with the most marked increases in unconjugated hyperbilirubinaemia and therefore the greatest risk of kernicterus are those associated with haemolysis in the newborn: (a) Feto-maternal blood group incompatibility; (b) Hereditary spherocytosis; (c) Red cell enzyme deficiency such as glucose-6-phosphate dehydrogenase deficiency.

The increased incidence of kernicterus in these conditions is thought to be due to raised haematin levels in blood which displaces bilirubin from albumin (Odell 1959).

**Kernicterus**

Kernicterus, the presence of unconjugated bilirubin in the basal ganglia at autopsy, was first described by Orth in 1875. Clinically, the term 'kernicterus' has been used to describe a syndrome of high-pitched cry, hypertonicity and opisthotonus followed by athetosis, asymmetric spasticity, hearing loss and dental anomalies. The association between neonatal hyperbilirubinaemia and yellow-stained basal ganglia at autopsy was observed by Mollison and Cutbush in 1949. If plasma unconjugated bilirubin in the newborn rises and remains elevated, the risk of kernicterus increases. The bilirubin molecules less tightly bound to albumin molecules can be displaced by competitive inhibition. This competitive uncoupling is facilitated by hypoxaemia, acidaemia, hypoglycaemia or sepsis with a rapid rise in bilirubin levels (Harper et al 1980). Unbound, unconjugated bilirubin free in plasma is lipophilic and easily penetrates cell membranes. It may cause severe cell damage by interrupting mitochondrial enzyme activities and oxidative phosphorylation, especially in the cells of the basal ganglia. The most common sequelae in children who survive kerniterus are sensorineural hearing impairment, choreo-athetosis, asymmetrical spasticity and varying degrees of intellectual impairment (Harper et al 1980).

The level of free bilirubin which causes kernicterus is variable. Although a level of total unconjugaed unconjugated bilirubin of 340$\mu$mol/1 (20 mg per cent) has been suggested as being a critical value (Hsia et al 1952), kernicterus has occurred in preterm infants who were hypoxic, acidotic, hypo-albuminaemic, hypoglycaemic or who were receiving certain drugs, at levels well below 340$\mu$mol/l (Keenan et al 1972). Levels of 600 to 700$\mu$mol/l (35 to 40 mg per cent) have been recorded in healthy full term infants with no neurological or intellectual sequelae at follow-up.

## Investigation of neonatal jaundice

After noting maternal history, pregnancy and parturition details and full clinical examination of the infant, initial investigation of neonatal jaundice normally includes the tests listed in Table 13.3. Further specialised investigations are performed if indicated.

**Table 13.3** Initial investigations for neonatal jaundice

1. Serum bilirubin concentration: conjugated, unconjugated
2. Haematological investigations: haemoglobin, total differential and white cell count, blood film.
   Glucose-6-phosphate dehydrogenase screen
3. Immunological investigations: ABO group; Coombs'—direct, indirect
4. Infection screen: swabs—eye, ear, nose, throat, and umbilicus; urine for microscopy and culture; blood culture; lumbar puncture; virus serology; serum immunoglobins

The simple tests in Table 13.3 should provide sufficient information as to the cause of the infant's jaundice and indicate whether it is due to excessive formation of bilirubin, impaired hepatic clearance or delayed faecal excretion. The cause of jaundice is of paramount importance, for the aetiology will indicate the appropriate treatment to interrupt the accumulation and facilitate elimination of bilirubin, thereby reducing the risk of kernicterus.

## Management of neonatal jaundice

Three techniques are used to treat neonatal unconjugated hyperbilirubinaemia.

*Exchange transfusion*

This may take the form of exchange with packed cells, whole blood or albumin in the form of purified plasma protein fraction, depending on the indication. Exchange transfusion with blood is appropriate for replacement of circulating neonatal erythrocytes which are undergoing rapid haemolysis and for removal of high circulating levels of bilirubin. The volume of exchange is usually equivalent to twice the infant's blood volume, that is 2 × 80 ml/kg, and this will effect 85 to 95 per cent exchange of the infant's cells with those of the donor.

*Phototherapy*

This is the commonest treatment employed to treat neonatal hyperbilirubinaemia. In the blue light wave length band, 425 to 475 nm, unconjugated bilirubin is decomposed to photo-oxidation products which have not yet been identified but are collectively called 'photobilirubins' (Lightner et al 1979). These are water-soluble, and hence less able to cross cell membranes. They are therefore less likely to be neurotoxic.

Serum bilirubin levels are also reduced by phototherapy because of the ability of phototherapy to shorten intestinal transit time. This is thought to be caused by a temporary state of lactose intolerance. The effect of shortened transit time is to reduce the enterohepatic circulation of bilirubin so reducing plasma levels and increasing excretion in faeces. Phototherapy used in conjunction with exchange transfusion in severely affected infants can reduce the number of exchange transfusions required. Neither exchange transfusion nor phototherapy is free from possible adverse effects. Poorly controlled exchange transfusion can cause hypovolaemic shock or heart failure. Phototherapy is biologically very powerful and clinical complications are well documented (Harper et al 1980). It has been suggested that intermittent phototherapy amounting to one fifth the normal dose may be adequate and no less efficient in treating neonatal hyperbilirubinaemia.

*Drugs*

Since one of the main aetiological factors in causing physiological jaundice is immaturity in liver enzyme conjugation systems, it is reasonable to expect known inducers of these enzymes to reduce neonatal hyperbilirubinaemia. Increased hepatic enzyme activity can be demonstrated in neonates (and adults) exposed to enzyme-inducing agents such as phenobarbitone (Kreek and Sleisenger 1968, Crigler and Gold 1966). Similarly, exposure of the fetus *in utero* to such agents administered to the mother has been demonstrated to cause induction of fetal hepatic enzymes in animal models, using barbiturates (Conney et al 1960) and halogenated herbicides (Berry et al 1976). Whether this response is possible in the human fetus has been the subject of some controversy. Phenobarbitone was first suspected to be of value in the treatment of neonatal jaundice when epileptic mothers taking the drug had babies with less jaundice (Trölle 1968a). One study (Draffen et al 1976) showed no increased liver enzyme activity whereas other studies showed that neonatal bilirubin levels could be reduced by maternal administration of phenobarbitone prophylactically for 14 days before delivery (Trölle 1968b, Halpin et al 1972, Valaes et al 1980).

Other agents purported to reduce bilirubin levels in the newborn are alcohol (Waltman et al 1969), heroin (Nathenson et al 1972), glutethimide and other stimulators of liver cell smooth endoplasmic reticulum. The enzyme induction effect of heroin also serves to protect against respiratory distress syndrome (Glass et al 1971).

Although phenobarbitone induces more ligandin (the cytoplasmic transport Y-protein in the liver cell) and causes a mitotic increase in the number of liver cells, the mechanism of action is thought to include increases in hepatic blood flow, bile flow, rate of bile salt synthesis, bile salt pool, endoplasmic reticulum, other enzymes and also altered metabolism and excretion of drugs (Reyes et al 1969).

The overall effect is to improve bilirubin conjugation and this has been corroborated by observations that patients with Gilbert's disease (congenital unconjugated hyperbilirubinaemia) excrete more of their bile pigment as diglucuronide conjugate when taking barbiturates (Goresky et al 1978), concomitant with a reduction in their serum bilirubin concentrations.

Prophylactic administration of phenobarbitone to the mother has therefore been shown to be effective but is rarely used because of its sedative action, and of suggestions that it might be teratogenic, even though this is not relevant in late pregnancy. If the drugs are used postnatally in conjunction with phototherapy the result is no better than with phototherapy alone (Valdes et al 1971). As the list of reported adverse effects of phototherapy grows, so the search for an alternative transplacental enzyme induction agent continues.

Antipyrine has been used in patients with Gilbert's disease to reduce unconjugated bilirubin levels (Orme et al 1974), and it has the advantage over phenobarbitone in that it has no sedative effects. In a recent study using antepartum antipyrine prophylactically, neonatal bilirubin levels were reduced by 40 per cent on average (Lewis and Friedman 1979). Further evaluation may cause obstetricians and paediatricians to consider wider use of drugs for prophylaxis or treatment of neonatal hyperbilirubinaemia.

## DRUGS ASSOCIATED WITH NEONATAL JAUNDICE

A large number of drugs have been said to cause neonatal hyperbilirubinaemia. Some have well proven associations and are cited with good reason. Some are infrequently mentioned but the association has been verified. Many are cited as a result of isolated or anecdotal observations which have never been verified.

### Glucose-6-phosphate dehydrogenase deficiency

One cause of neonatal jaundice well documented to be associated with drug use is glucose-6-phosphate dehydrogenase (G-6-PD) deficiency. This enzyme is responsible for the first step of the pentose phosphate shunt, the alternative pathway for the catabolism of glucose. Certain drugs and some metabolic disturbances may precipitate haemolysis in individuals deficient in the enzyme.

G-6-PD deficiency is genetically determined and transmitted by a gene located on the X-chromosome. Full expression of the gene therefore occurs more frequently in the male, but great variability with respect to partial expression of the defect may be seen in the heterozygous female. Diagnosis can be made quickly and easily in most well equipped haematology departments using an enzyme assay technique.

The incidence and severity of the disease and the precipitating agents differ with race and ethnic group. Hyperbilirubinaemia in the neonate and subsequent kernicterus have frequently been observed in the newborn deficient in G-6-PD (Smith and Vella 1960).

The deficiency is widely distributed throughout the world. Among Caucasians the incidence is greatest in the Mediterranean area. Thirty per cent of males in some areas of Sardinia are deficient in the enzyme. It also occurs with high frequency among Greeks, Iranians and Sephardic Jews. Among Mongolian groups Chinese, Malays, Philippinos and Indonesians are known to be affected. In black American males the incidence is said to be 9 to 13 per cent and in black American females 2 to 4 per cent (Tarlov et al 1962). In Africa the incidence is higher in those areas where falciparum malaria is endemic, involving 25 per cent of the population. The deficiency is said to protect against intracellular invasion by the malaria parasite; so-called 'balanced pleomorphism'.

The heterogenicity of this deficiency is reflected in various degrees of enzyme deficiency, the type of drugs necessary to produce haemolysis, the type of cells in the body affected by the deficiency and the susceptibility to neonatal jaundice. Theoretically, it is possible that all drugs which cause haemolysis in G-6-PD deficient individuals can precipitate jaundice in the susceptible newborn if administered to the mother in sufficient doses at or near term. In this category sulphonamides and nitrofurantoin are likely to be most commonly used. Pregnant mothers of G-6-PD deficient babies can have a pica resulting in ingestion of naphthalene-containing compounds such as moth balls. This can cause a haemolytic episode in the newborn (Zinkham and Childs 1958).

Drugs reported to have produced haemolysis in G-6-PD deficient individuals are shown in Table IV, and use of these agents should be avoided in susceptible patients.

**Table 13.4** Drugs capable of introducing haemolytic anaemia in glucose-6-phosphate dehydrogenase deficiency

| | | |
|---|---|---|
| Acetanilide | Menadiol | Sulphamethoxazole |
| Acetysalicylic acid | Methylene Blue | Sulphamerazine |
| *p*-Aminobenzoic acid | Nalidixic acid | Sulphadimidine |
| Aminophenol | Naphthalene | Sulphafurazole |
| Aniline | Neoarsphenamine | Sulphamethizole |
| Antazoline | Nitrofurantoin | Sulphadimethoxine |
| Antipyrine | Nitrofurazone | Sulphathiazole |
| Ascorbic acid | Primaquine | Sulphamethoxydiazine |
| Chloramphenicol | Pentaquine | Sulphapyridine |
| Chloroquine | Phenacetin | Sulphaphenazole |
| Co-trimoxazole | Phenylhydrazine | Sulphamethoxypyridazine |
| Dapsone | Probenecid | Sulfadoxine |
| Dimercaprol | Procainamide | Sulfametopyrazine |
| Diphenhydramine | Pyrimethamine | Sodium nitrate |
| Fava beans (broad beans) | Quinidine | Thiazosulphone |
| Furaltadone | Quinine | Trinitrotoluene |
| Furazolidone | Quinocide | Tripelennamine |
| Hydroxychloroquine | Sulphasalazine | Vitamin K |
| Mepacrine | Sulphacetamide | |

## Agents competing for albumin binding sites

*Sulphonamides.* In addition to their role in G-6-PD deficient individuals, sulphonamides can make neonatal jaundice more dangerous. Silverman et al (1956) first noted an association between the administration of the antibiotic sulfisoxazole to preterm infants, and the occurrence of kernicterus at low levels of total serum bilirubin. Odell (1959) demonstrated that this was due to competitive displacement of bilirubin bound at the secondary 'low affinity' binding site on the albumin molecule. Since that time many endogenous and exogenous water-soluble organic ions have been identified as competitors for binding to albumin. These effectively decrease the power of plasma to sequester bilirubin in a safer form, or increase the dissociation of bilirubin from albumin with liberation of free unconjugated bilirubin, which is diffusible and toxic (Hagberg et al 1975).

Examples of endogenous substances which compete for albumin binding sites are non-esterified fatty acids (Wooley and Hunter 1970) and haematin. Haematin from breakdown of haemoglobin is present in increased amounts in haemolytic conditions. Its presence affords a ready explanation for the higher risk of kernicterus in haemolytic as compared to non-haemolytic hyperbilirubinaemias.

Exogenous substances like some sulphonamides, salicylates (Broderson 1974) and benzoates have a similar effect. A provisional list of the displacing effect of 150 drugs tested *in vitro* has been published (Brodersen 1978).

Ideally all drugs intended for use in the neonate or in pregnant or lactating women, should be tested for displacing effect (Stern 1972). If any of the drugs implicated are to be considered for therapeutic use in late pregnancy or the newborn, a few guidelines may be of practical value for the clinician.

Drugs which are given in low doses such as hormones, digoxin and highly effective diuretics are safe to use since the molar amount of the drug required to occupy a significant fraction of the reserve albumin is unlikely to be reached. Cationic drugs and most electroneutral substances such as gentamicin, antihistamines, general anasthetics and benzodiazepines are not bound competively at the binding site. The effect of sulphonamides is variable. Sulphadiazine is the weakest competitor for albumin binding and possibly safe at usual doses. Analgesic and anti-inflammatory agents such as salicylates are potent competitors. The highest degrees of displacement are seen with radiographic contrast media. These are given in high doses and occupy the reserve albumin very efficiently.

Dissociation of bilirubin from albumin is favoured by certain metabolic conditions such as hypothermia and hypoglycaemia in which plasma non-esterified fatty acids are increased. Acidosis (Stern and Denton 1965) and hypoxia (Lucey et al 1964) also favour dissociation. Hypo-albuminaemia by its very nature reduces the number of possible binding sites and favours elevated free unconjugated bilirubin in plasma.

**Drugs causing jaundice by prehepatic effects**

*Vitamin K.* In addition to the association of vitamin K with jaundice in G-6-PD deficient individuals Lucey and Dolan (1959) observed that administration of large doses (72 mg) of the water soluble synthetic vitamin K analogue menadione sodium bisulphite to mothers in labour was associated with early marked hyperbilirubinaemia in preterm infants. It was not established in this study if the mechanism of jaundice was one of hepatic toxicity or haemolysis, although other workers have observed haemolytic anaemia in preterm infants following large doses of water soluble vitamin K analogues (Gasser 1953). Fortunately the dose required for prophylaxis against haemorrhagic disease of the newborn is measured in micrograms, so that safe and effective use of these drugs is possible.

Vitamin $K_1$ (phytomenadione), the naturally occurring compound in our diet, has not been implicated. Vitamin $K_2$ (menaquinone) is formed by bacteria in the intestine. Thus, use of vitamin $K_1$

or of low doses of the synthetic analogue vitamin $K_3$ (menaphthone), 1 mg of the sodium bisulphite complex administered directly to the baby orally, can be recommended.

*Thiazides*. These have been reported to cause jaundice through haemolysis in newborn who are not deficient in glucose-6-phosphate dehygrogenase. Two possible cases were observed by Harley et al (1964).

## Drugs causing jaundice by hepatic effects

Many drugs have been suggested to have an effect at the stage of conjugation of bilirubin in the liver. Alcohol, antipyrine, dicophane, heroin and phenobarbitone have all been shown to reduce bilirubin levels by inducing the hepatic enzyme systems involved in bilirubin clearance. Other drugs may interfere with conjugation and precipitate jaundice.

The antibiotic novobiocin is a potent inhibitor of glucuronidation (Hargreaves and Holton 1962), its action being mediated by competition for uridine diphosphate-glucuronyl transferase. Other drugs like streptomycin and chloramphenicol can be shown to have a similar effect *in vitro* (Waters et al 1958). The only clinical correlation which has been established with certainty is with novobiocin, which has been found to produce jaundice in newborn humans (Sutherland and Keller 1961).

It would be prudent where reasonable to avoid the use of drugs in labour and neonatal life which have been shown to depend upon the same uptake and conjugation sites as bilirubin. As a result, if chloramphenicol is used in the newborn blood levels arc closely monitored to avoid toxic levels of drug concentration in plasma.

## Drugs causing jaundice by posthepatic effects

The reports of an increased incidence of jaundice in infants whose mothers received phenothiazine tranquillisers during labour (Jones 1964, John 1975) have not been substantiated in studies by a number of authors including Done (1964), Fitzgerald et al (1963) and Drew and Kitchen (1976). In the work of Done (1964) and Fitzgerald et al (1963) negative results were also found with erythromycin, oxytetracycline, pethidine and scopolamine. Drew and Kitchen (1976) also failed to show any effect on neonatal jaundice of general anaesthesia (atropine, thiopentone, succinylcholine, tubocurarine, nitrous oxide and oxygen), local anaesthesia, ampicillin, penicillin, and sulphadimidine when these agents were administered to the mother before delivery.

Ganglion-blocking drugs like hexamethonium used in pregnancy hypertension can cause paralytic ileus in the newborn. As a result of intestinal stasis there is an increased enterohepatic circulation of bile salts in the infant and raised serum bilirubin levels (Morris 1953, Hallum and Hatchuel 1954).

**Drugs causing jaundice by unknown mechanisms**

Maternal administration of diazepam has been reported to cause an increased incidence of jaundice in infants (McIntosh 1970) and this finding was confirmed by Drew and Kitchen (1976). No theoretical basis for its mechanism of action is known. Schiff et al (1971) suggested that diazepam caused displacement of bilirubin from albumin in addition, a dangerous combination of actions. It seems likely that when the drug is given parenterally, it is the benzoate preservative which causes displacement, and not diazepam itself. The risk is very small, since in a recent study 10 mg of diazepam given intravenously just before delivery produced no significant increase in hyperbilirubinaemia (McAllister 1980). When considering the use of diazepam it would be wise to adopt the recommendation of Kanto et al (1974). In view of the wide variations in the metabolism and excretion of diazepam by the neonate, doses higher than 10 to 20 mg were not recommended for the mother during labour on the grounds that competitive inhibition of the conjugation might lead to hyperbilirubinaemia.

Friedman et al (1978) concluded that epidural anaesthesia contributed to an increased incidence of neonatal jaundice. Bupivacaine, the amide frequently used in epidural anaesthesia, is known to cross the placenta and is metabolised in the liver where some of its metabolites are glucuronidated. *In vitro*, no effect could be demonstrated on the capacity of the liver microsomes to conjugate bilirubin (Friedman and Lewis 1978). If an association with epidural anaesthesia really exists, the mechanism of induction of neonatal hyperbilirubinaemia remains unexplained.

Hormones are also of relevance in neonatal jaundice. Babies with congenital hypothyroidism (Åkerrén 1955) and babies of diabetic mothers (Taylor et al 1963) are known to be prone to neonatal jaundice, and other endocrine causes have been implicated.

The increased frequency of neonatal jaundice associated with infants that are breast fed in comparison to formula fed babies was first reported by Newman and Gross in 1963. The inhibition of glucuronyl transferase activity by pregnenediol secreted in milk was suggested to be a cause by Arias et al (1964). This theory proved to be unsatisfactory, since milks with strong inhibitory properties contained minimal quantities of the hormone. Later research showed that the inhibition of glucuronyl transferase activity was not hormonal but rather caused by free fatty acids, especially linoleic acid (Horiguchi and Bauer 1975). Those milks with the greatest capacity for inhibition of glucuronidation contain the largest amounts of lipase (and hence free fatty acids) even at low temperatures, which explains why stored milks retain inhibitory properties. When treating breast milk jaundice substitution of dried milk usually effects a decreased in plasma bilirubin in the newborn within 48 hours.

Use of drugs such as novobiocin or some sulphonamides which are known to be hazardous in the neonate, causing jaundice or potentiating adverse effects of jaundice, should be avoided in late pregnancy. Other drugs, where the evidence regarding their causative association with neonatal jaundice is inconclusive, can usually be avoided if suitable alternatives are available.

*Oxytocin*

Maternal oxytocin administration in labour and its role in the aetiology of neonatal jaundice has been the subject of much discussion, especially in the British literature. Ghosh and Hudson (1972) studied a series of 197 births. There was a significant increase in neonatal jaundice in infants born of mothers who received oxytocin for either induction or acceleration of labour. They suggested that oxytocin might interfere with hepatic conjugation of bilirubin. The gestation of these babies was not clear but all weighed over 5 lbs (2200 g). In 1973 Davies et al reported a prospective study which supported Ghosh and Hudson's (1972) findings. All 78 babies studied were full term. They suggested that the jaundice was due to decreased cord serum cortisol levels in babies delivered following induced labour. The absence of the normal endogenous cortisol spurt in such labours, might cause a delay in maturation of hepatic enzyme systems. They considered that it was possible that oxytocin might not be causing the jaundice directly, the interruption of pregnancy itself being responsible.

Roberts and Weaver, in 1974, also found an association between oxytocin and neonatal jaundice in a review of 215 births with birthweights over 2500 g. They pointed out that neonatal jaundice following oxytocin therapy was a minor problem in comparison to the possible consequences of prolonged labour if oxytocin was witheld; intra-uterine anoxia, neonatal hypoxia, and cerebral damage could result.

Opposing views came from two prospective studies (Gould et al 1974, Gray and Mitchell 1974), and one large retrospective study from America, (Friedman and Sachtleben 1974) which failed to show any significant association between oxytocin and neonatal jaundice following spontaneous, accelerated or induced labours.

Calder et al (1974), in a prospective study, concurred with the findings of Davies et al (1973), stating that an association existed and theorised that the mechanism was one of premature interruption of pregnancy which caused the jaundice, and not the drug itself. A much larger prospective study by Beazley and Alderman (1975) failed to demonstrate any significant difference in incidence of neonatal jaundice following spontaneous, oxytocin-induced or augmented labours. On the other hand, they did find a significant dose-dependant relationship between mean total dose of oxytocin and the incidence of neonatal jaundice. Subsequently, three large retrospective studies (Chalmers et al 1975, Campbell et al 1975, Sims and Neligan 1975) again supported the theory that premature interruption of pregnancy and not oxytocin, caused the jaundice.

In 1976 Friedman and Sachtleben found that the incidence of jaundice correlated not with oxytocin use but with mid-forceps and breech extraction, suggesting that trauma from operative delivery following induction of labour was an important factor. Prospective studies by Beazley and Weekes (1976) and Chew and Swann (1977) disagreed with each other in their conclusions. Chew and Swann (1977), while quoting significantly higher mean bilirubin concentrations in oxytocin-induced labours, agreed with Beazley and Weekes (1976) with respect to the failure to demonstrate any dose-dependant relationship, in contrast to Beazley and Alderman's (1975) observations.

The major studies quoted above together with other work are thus difficult to assess. Large retrospective studies and smaller prospective studies not only vary in the level of serum bilirubin concentration accepted as being hyperbilirubinaemic but also differ in their conclusions. In selecting groups to be compared, some workers used gestational age, while others used birth weight. Not all the studies involved matching for gestational age, and in many no allowance was made for other variables such as epidural anaesthesia, known to be associated with an increased incidence of neonatal jaundice (Friedman et al 1978).

Until recently, no mechanism which explained how oxytocin might directly cause hyperbilirubinaemia has been advanced. Inhibition of glucuronidation by oxytocin could not be demonstrated *in vitro* by Friedman and Lewis (1978), unlike novobiocin. A possible explanation for an effect of oxytocin in the aetiology of neonatal jaundice has now appeared. Singhi and Singh (1979) observed that serum osmolarity and sodium concentrations are significantly reduced in infants delivered of mothers who received oxytocin in labour. This antidiuretic action of oxytocin, similar to that of the other posterior pituitary hormone vasopressin, was confirmed by Buchan (1979). He showed that the resultant osmotic swelling leads to decreased deformability of erythrocytes and hence more rapid destruction in the reticulo-endothelial system, with resultant hyperbilirubinaemia in the neonate. This explanation lends some weight to the inconclusive evidence implicating oxytocin in the aetiology of neonatal jaundice.

Oxytocin is a safe, cost-effective drug of proved efficacy and only a simple recommendation to keep to the minimum dose required for a desired response suffices; a recommendation which applies to any drug.

## REFERENCES

Åkerrén Y 1955 Early diagnosis and early therapy in congenital cretinism. Archives of Disease in Childhood 30: 254–256

Arias I M Gartner L M, Seifter S, Furman M 1964 Prolonged neonatal unconjugated hyperbilirubinaemia associated with breast feeding and a steroid pregnane-3(alpha), 20(beta)-diol in maternal milk that inhibits glucuronide formation in vitro. Journal of Clinical Investigation 43: 2037–2047

Beazley J M, Alderman B 1975 Neonatal hyperbilirubinaemia following the use of oxytocin in labour. British Journal of Obstetrics and Gynaecology 82: 265–271

Beazley J M, Weekes A R 1976. Neonatal hyperbilirubinaemia following the use of prostaglandin $E_2$ in labour. British Journal of Obstetrics and Gynaecology 83: 62–67

Berry D L, Zachariah P K, Namkung M J, Juchau M R 1976 Transplacental induction of carcinogen-hydroxylating systems with 2,3,7,8,-tetrachlorodibenzo-*p*-dioxin. Toxicology and Applied Pharmacology 36: 569–584

Bratteby L E, Garby L, Wadman B 1968 Studies on erythrokinetics in infancy. Acta paediatrica Scandinavica 57: 305–310

Broderson R 1974 Competitive binding of bilirubin and drugs to human serum albumin, studied by enzymatic oxidation. Journal of Clinical Investigation 54: 1353–1364

Broderson R 1978 Free bilirubin in blood plasma of the newborn: Effects of albumin, fatty acids, pH displacing drugs and phototherapy. In: Stern L, Oh W, Friis-Hansen B (editors) Intensive case in the newborn II. Masson, New York, pp. 331–346

Brown A K 1962 Neonatal jaundice. Pediatric Clinics of North America, 9: 575–603

Buchan P C 1979 Pathogenesis of neonatal hyperbilirubinaemia after induction of labour with oxytocin. British Medical Journal. ii: 1255–1257

Calder A A, Moar V A, Ounsted M K, Turnbull A C 1974 Increased bilirubin levels in neonates after induction of labour by intravenous prostaglandin $E_2$ or oxytocin. Lancet ii: 1339–1342

Campbell N, Harvey D, Norman A P 1975 Increased frequency of neonatal jaundice in a maternity hospital, British Medical Journal ii: 548–552

Chalmers J, Campbell H, Turnbull A C 1975 Use of oxytocin and incidence of neonatal jaundice. British Medical Journal ii: 116–118

Chew W C, Swann I L 1977 Influence of simultaneous low amniotomy and oxytocin infusion and other maternal factors on neonatal jaundice: a prospective study. British Medical Journal i: 72–73

Conney A H, Davidson C, Gastel R Burns J J 1960 Adaptive increases in drug metabolising enzymes induced by phenobarbital and other drugs. Journal of Pharmacology and Experimental Therapeutics 130: 1–8

Crigler J F, Gold N I 1966 Sodium phenobarbital induced decrease in serum bilirubin in an infant with congenital non haemolytic jaundice and kernicterus. Journal of Clinical Investigation. 45: 998–999

Davies D P, Gomersall R, Robertson R, Gray Q P Turnbull A C 1973 Neonatal jaundice and maternal oxytocin infusion. British Medical Journal iii: 476–477

Done A J 1964 Developmental pharmacology. Clinical Pharmacology and Therapeutics 5: 432–479

Draffen G H, Dollery C T, Davies D S, Krauer B, Williams F M, Clare R A, Trudinger B J, Darling M. Sertel H, Hawkins D F 1976 Maternal and neonatal elimination of amobarbital after treatment of the mother with barbiturates during late pregnancy. Clinical Pharmacology and Therapeutics 19: 271–275

Drew J H, Kitchen W H 1976 The effect of maternally administered drugs on bilirubin concentrations in the newborn infant. Journal of Pediatrics 89: 657–661

Felsher B F, Maidman J E, Carpio N M, Couvering K V, Woolley M M 1978 Reduced hepatic bilirubin uridine disphosphate glucuronyl transferase and uridine diphosphate glucose dehydrogenase activity in the human fetus. Pediatric Research 12: 838–840

Fitzgerald W J, Pahl I, Hall L, Mella R 1963 The influence of propiomazine on neonatal serum bilirubin levels. Obstetrics and Gynaecology. 22: 709–712

Friedman E A, Sachtleben M R 1974 Oxytocin and neonatal jaundice. Lancet ii: 600

Friedman E A, Sachtleben M R 1976 Neonatal jaundice in association with oxytocin stimulation of labour and operative delivery. British Medical Journal i: 198–199

Friedman L A, Lewis P J 1978 Maternal drug therapy and neonatal jaundice. In: Lewis P J (editor) Therapeutic problems in pregnancy. Lancaster, MTP Press, pp. 141, 141–151.

Friedman L, Lewis P J, Clifton P, Bulpitt C 1978 Factors influencing the incidence of neonatal jaundice. British Medical Journal i: 1235–1237

Gasser C 1953 Die haemolytische Frühgeburtenänamie mit spontaner Innenkörperbilding ein neues syndrom beobachter am 14 Fällen. Helvetica Paediatrica Acta 8: 491–529

Ghosh A, Hudson F P 1972 Oxytocin agents and neonatal hyperbilirubinaemia. Lancet ii: 823

Glass L, Rajegowda B K, Evans H E 1971 Absence of respiratory distress syndrome in premature infants of heroin addicted mothers. Lancet ii: 685–686

Goresky C A, Gordon E R, Shaffer E A, Paré P, Carrasavas D, Arnoff A 1978. Definition of a conjugation of dysfunction in Gilbert's syndrome: studies of the handling of bilirubin loads and the pattern of bilirubin conjugate secreted in bile. Clinical Science and Molecular Medicine 55: 63–71

Gould S R, Mountrose U, Brown D J, Whitehouse W L, Barnardon D E 1974 Influence of previous contraception and maternal oxytocin infusion on neonatal jaundice. British Medical Journal iii: 228–231

Gray H G, Mitchell R 1974 Neonatal hyperbilirubinaemia and oxytocin. Lancet ii: 1144

Hagberg B, Hagberg G, Olow I 1975 The changing panorama of cerebral palsy in Sweden, 1954–1970. I Analysis of the general changes. Acta paediatrica Scandinavica 64: 187–192. II Analysis of the various syndromes. Acta paediatrica Scandinavica 64: 193–200

Hallum J L, Hatchuel W l F 1954 Congenital paralytic ileus in a premature baby as a complication of hexamethonium bromide therapy for toxaemia of pregnancy.

Archives of Disease in Childhood 29: 354–356
Halpin T F, Jones A R, Bishop H L, Lerner S 1972 Prophylaxis of neonatal hyperbilirubinaemia with phenobarbital. Obstetrics and Gynaecology 40: 85–90
Hargreaves T, Holton J B 1962. Jaundice of the newborn due to novobiocin. Lancet i: 839
Harley J D, Robin H, Robertson S E J 1964 Thiazide induced neonatal haemolysis. British Medical Journal i: 696–697
Harper R G, Sia C G, Kierney C M P 1980 Kernicterus 1980: problems and practices viewed from the perspective of the practicing clinician. Clinics in Perinatalogy 7(1): 75–92
Horiguchi T, Bauer C 1975 Ethnic difference in neonatal jaundice comparison of Japanese and Caucasian newborn infants. American Journal of Obstetrics and Gynaecology. 121: 71–74
Hsia D Y–Y, Allen F H, Gellis S S, Diamond L K 1952 Erythroblastosis fetalis VIII. Studies of serum bilirubin in relation to kernicterus. New England Journal of Medicine 247: 668–671
Jacobsen J 1969 Binding of bilirubin to human serum albumin; determination of the dissociation constants. Federation of European Biochemical Societies Letter 5: 112–114
John E 1975 Promazine and neonatal hyperbilirubinaemia. Medical Journal of Australia ii: 342–344
Jones B 1964 Glucuronyl transferase inhibition by steroids. Journal of Pediatrics 64: 815–821
Kanto J, Erkkola R, Sellman R 1974 Perinatal metabolism of diazepam. British Medical Journal i: 641–642
Keenan W J, Perlstein P H, Light I J, Sutherland J M 1972 Kernicterus in small, sick, preterm infants receiving phototherapy. Pediatrics 49: 652–655
Kreek M J, Sleisenger M H 1968 Reduction of serum unconjugated bilirubin with phenobarbitone in adult congenital non-haemolytic unconjugated hyperbilirubinaemia. Lancet ii: 73 –78
Levi A J, Gatmaitan Z, Arias I M 1969 Two hepatic cytoplasmic protein fractions Y and Z, and their possible role in the hepatic uptake of bilirubin, sulphobromophthalein and other anions. Journal of Clinical Investigation 48: 2156–2167
Lewis P J, Friedman L A 1979 Prophylaxis of neonatal jaundice with maternal antipyrine treatment. Lancet i: 300–302
Lightner D A, Wooldridge T A, McDonagh A F 1979 Photobilirubin : an early bilirubin photoproduct detected by absorbance difference spectroscopy. Proceedings of the National Academy of Sciences of the United States of America 76 : 29–32
Lucey J F, Dolan R G 1959 Hyperbilirubinaemia of newborn infants associated with the parenteral administration of a Vitamin K analogue to the mothers. Pediatrics 23: 553–560
Lucey J F, Hibbard E, Behrman R E, Esquivel De Gardo F O, Windle W F 1964 Kernicterus in asphyxiated newborn rhesus monkeys. Experimental Neurology 9: 43–58
Luzeau R, Levillain P Odievre M, Lemonniare A 1974 Demonstration of a lipolytic activity in human milk that inhibits the glucuro-conjugation of bilirubin. Biomedicine 21: 258–262
McAllister C B 1980 Placental transfer and neonatal effects of diazepam when administered to women just before delivery. British Journal of Anaesthesia 52: 423–427
McIntosh A 1970 Hyperbilirubinaemia in neonates. Medical Journal of Australia ii: 101–102
Mollison P L, Cutbush M 1949 Haemolytic disease of the newborn. Criteria of severity. British Medical Journal i: 123–130

Morris N 1953 Hexamethonium compounds in the treatment of pre-eclampsia and essential hypertension during pregnancy. Lancet i: 322–324
Nathenson G, Cohen M I, Litt I F, McNamara H 1972 The effect of maternal heroin addiction on neonatal jaundice. Journal of Pediatrics 81: 899–903
Newman A J, Gross S 1963 Hyperbilirubinaemia in breast fed infants. Pediatrics 32: 995–1001
Odell G B 1959 The dissociation of bilirubin from albumin and its clinical implications. Journal of Pediatrics 55: 268–279
Odell G B, Cukier J O, Maglalang A C 1976 Pathogenesis of neonatal hyperbilirubinaemia. In: Young D S, Hicks J M editors) The neonate. Wiley, New York, pp. 171–184
Orme M L E, Davies L, Breckenridge A 1974 Increased glucuronidation of bilirubin in man and rat by administration of antipyrine (phenazone). Clinical Sciences and Molecular Medicine 40: 511–518
Reyes H, Levi A J, Gatmaitan Z, Arais I M 1969 Organic anion binding protein in rat liver. Drug induction and its physiologic consequence. Proceedings of the National Academy of Sciences of the United States of America 64: 168–170
Roberts L, Weaver A 1974 Labour and neonatal jaundice. Lancet i: 935
Schenker S, Dawber N H, Schmid R 1964 Bilirubin metabolism in the fetus. Journal of Clinical Investigation 43: 32–39
Schiff D, Chan G, Stern L 1971 Fixed drug combinations and the displacement of bilirubin from albumin. Pediatrics 48: 139–141
Silverman W A, Anderson D H, Blanc W A, Crozier D N 1956 A difference in mortality rate and incidence of kernicterus among premature infants allocated to two prophylactic antibiotic regimens. Pediatrics 18: 614–625
Sims D G, Neligan G A 1975 Factors affecting the increased incidence of severe non-haemolytic neonatal jaundice. British Journal of Obstetrics and Gynaecology 82: 863–867
Singhi S, Singh M 1979 Pathogenesis of oxytocin induced neonatal hyperbilirubinaemia. Archives of Disease in Childhood 54: 400–402
Smith G D, Vella F 1960 Erythrocyte enzyme deficiency in unexplained kernicterus. Lancet i: 1133–1134
Stern L 1972 Drug Interactions, Part II. Drugs, the newborn infant and the binding of bilirubin to albumin. Pediatrics 49: 916–918
Stern L, Denton R L 1965 Kernicterus in small premature infants. Pediatrics 35: 483–485
Stern L, Kanna N N, Levy G, Yaffe S J 1970. Effect of phenobarbital on hyperbilirubinaemia and glucuronide formation in newborns. American Journal of Disease in Childhood 120: 26–31
Sutherland J M, Keller W H 1961. Novobiocin and neonatal hyperbilirubinaemia. An investigation of the relationship in an epidemic of neonatal hyperbilirubinaemia. American Journal of Diseases of Children 101: 447–453
Takimoto M, Matsuda I 1971 β-glycuronidase activity in the stool of the newborn infant. Biology of the Neonate 18: 66–70
Tarlov A R, Brewer G J, Carson P E, Alving A S 1962 Primaquine sensitivity. Archives of Internal Medicine 109: 137–162
Taylor P M, Wolfson J H, Bright N H, Birchard E L, Derinoz E M, Watson D W 1963 Hyperbilirubinaemia in infants of diabetic mothers. Biology of the Neonate 5: 289–298
Trölle D 1968a Phenobarbitone and neonatal icterus Lancet i: 251–252
Trölle D 1968b Decrease of total serum bilirubin concentration in newborn infants after phenobarbitone treatment. Lancet ii: 705–708
Valaes T, Kipouros R, Petmazaki S, Solman M, Doxiadis S A 1980 Effectiveness and safety of prenatal phenobarbital for the prevention of neonatal jaundice. Pediatric Research 14: 947–952
Valdes O S, Maurer H M Shumway C N, Draper D A, Hossaini A A 1971 Controlled clinical trial of phenobarbital and/or light in reducing neonatal

hyperbilirubinaemia in a predominantly negro population. Journal of Pediatrics 79: 1015–1017

Waltman R, Bonura F, Nigrin G, Pipat C 1969 Ethanol and neonatal bilirubin levels. Lancet ii: 108

Waters W J, Dunham R, Bowan W R 1958 Inhibition of bilirubin conjugation *in vitro*. Proceedings of the Society for Experimental Biology and Medicine 99: 175–177

Wooley P V, Hunter M J 1970 Binding and circular dichroism data on bilirubin—albumin in the presence of oleate and salicylate. Archives of Biochemistry and Biophysics 140: 197–209

Zinkham W H, Childs B 1958 A defect of glutathione metabolites in erythrocytes from patients with naphthalene induced hemolytic anaemia. Pediatrics 22: 461–471

# Drugs and breast feeding

## INTRODUCTION

The proportion of women who elect to breast feed their infants is increasing both in this country and in developing countries. A survey in Cambridge is typical; 51 per cent of babies in 1976 were breast fed at birth compared to 39 per cent in 1971 (Whichlow 1979). Among the many factors which influence the mother's decision to breast feed is the medical advice she receives during her pregnancy. Following recognition of certain objective advantages of breast feeding, it is now considered good medical practice actively to encourage women to breast feed their infants, always provided the encouragement falls some way short of active persuasion and that those women who do not breast feed do not feel a sense of rejection or disapproval.

There are two aspects to the subject of drugs and breast feeding. First, drug treatment in the puerperium can be used to influence lactation directly, either suppressing it or augmenting it. Secondly, passage of drugs into breast milk can give rise to difficulties when treating women who are breast feeding their infants.

## DRUGS AND THE CONTROL OF LACTATION

### Normal lactation

During pregnancy the circulating levels of the anterior pituitary hormone prolactin begin to rise in the first trimester and increase progressively to reach a peak level before delivery some 10 to 50 times greater than those in the non-pregnant state (Tyson et al 1972, Rigg et al 1977). Despite this, full lactation does not occur until some 36 to 48 hours after delivery because the high levels of circulating oestrogen and progesterone, present at the end of pregnancy, block the lactogenic effect of prolactin on the mammary tissue. With delivery of the placenta this progesterone and oestrogen block is removed and prolactin is free to stimulate lactation.

Although these hormone effects are important, they are outweighed by the effects of suckling, the most powerful determinant of lactation. It should be remembered that even an adopting mother can lactate and feed an infant if the child can be persuaded to suckle the breast persistently. Suckling markedly stimulates the release of both prolactin and oxytocin, promoting lactation and milk expression. In addition, active suckling empties the breast of milk and directly encourages further lactation.

**Promotion of lactation**

It appears that the most important factors for the establishment of successful feeding are the motivation and confidence of the mother; hormonal factors are of secondary importance. Motivation can be aided by giving the pregnant woman an explanation of the main advantages of breast feeding. Apart from the psychological benefits which mothers may derive from the close contact with their infants, there are certain advantages of breast feeding which can be objectively defended. These are in brief:

1. The fats, proteins, minerals and sugars in human milk are more suitable for the growth and development of the human infant than are those in cow's milk.
2. Feeding of cow's milk to an infant increases the likelihood that it will suffer from eczema and asthma.
3. Breast fed infants suffer far fewer gastrointestinal infections than do bottle fed infants.
4. Breast feeding confers some protection to the mother against breast cancer in later life.

Many women having initiated breast feeding abandon it early, claiming that they have insufficient milk and fearing that their child is not being adequately fed. The fact that some enthusiastic clinicians can achieve a very high incidence of successful breast feeding in their patients, tends to suggest that regimens which maintain the mother's confidence to succeed are extremely important. The key to success in these regimens seems to be constant assurance and interest on the part of the woman's attendants.

Drug treatment of inadequate or failing lactation seems to have little place. Several drugs are known to increase prolactin secretion and, in theory, these might be effective promotors of lactation. Synthetic thyrotropin-releasing hormone (TRH) stimulates prolactin release, and attempts have been made to enhance lactational performance in women by treatment with TRH, but the results are equivocal. TRH administration has promoted breast engorgement with rises in both milk volume and milk fat composition (Tyson et al 1975, 1976) and restored full nursing in women with lactational insufficiency (Zanartu et al 1975). In contrast, other studies detected no effect of TRH on milk yield or composition in normal women (Zarate et al 1976, Canales et al 1977, Hall and Kay 1977), suggesting that in women prolactin secretion is not usually rate-limiting. TRH has also been used to restart lactation in women with premature infants whose milk secretion had earlier been suppressed with bromocriptine (Canales et al 1977).

Various other drugs also increase prolactin secretion, although few have as marked an effect as does suckling itself. Metoclopramide is an anti-emetic drug, whose action depends on it being a dopamine receptor agonist with a predominantly central site of action. Metoclopramide certainly causes prolactin release (McNeilly et al 1974) and there is some indication that this drug can cause increased milk production in women (Sonson 1975). The use of metoclopramide in women with a past history of defective lactation resulted in an increase in prolactin concentrations as well as an improvement in milk yield (Guzman et al 1979). A double blind placebo-controlled trial of this drug, in a dose of 10 mg 3 times a day for one week, in women attempting to breast feed following caesarean section, had the interesting result that all 10 women treated with the active drugs succeeded in establishing breast feeding (Lewis et al 1980), but all 10 women treated with placebo under identical double blind circumstances also succeeded in establishing breast feeding. These results suggest that the placebo effect is very great in breast feeding and that confidence, encouragement and individual care are the important determinants.

## Suppression of lactation

Unfortunately, drugs are more often required for the suppression of lactation in women who do not wish to breast feed than for the enhancement of lactation.

Natural suppression will occur without the use of drugs and depends only on the exclusion of suckling. If no milk is removed from the breast, then lactation will eventually cease. The disadvantage of this simple method is that the breasts may become sore and tender. Pain usually occurs 3 or 4 days after delivery but seldom extends beyond the first week. Supportive clothing and simple analgesics may be used to relieve the discomfort. Since natural suppression is always effective, the use of drugs to suppress lactation can only be justified if they significantly reduce this breast discomfort. Some authorities claim that the discomfort is really minimal and that the use of drugs for suppression of lactation is a dangerous extravagance. There is no doubt from placebo-controlled trials that a placebo is effective in the relief of breast discomfort following withdrawal of suckling.

Oestrogens were first used in lactation suppression in 1938 (Foss and Phillips 1938). It is interesting that in the original paper describing the use of oestrogen, almost all the women so treated were having their lactation suppressed following a stillbirth. Oestrogens were used almost universally for suppressing lactation until it was realised that, apart from their relative ineffectiveness, they have major unwanted side effects. All prolong the period of bloody discharge from the puerperal uterus and they significantly predispose the woman to thrombo-embolism in the puerperium (Daniel et al 1967), probably by increasing synthesis of various clotting factors. The puerperium is a period of high risk for thrombo-embolism anyway and relatively large doses of oestrogen have to be used in order to suppress lactation effectively. If oestrogen is not given within the first 24 hours after delivery, initiation of lactation cannot be suppressed. Furthermore, the treatment has to be prolonged for at least 14 days. Many different oestrogens have been used, the most convenient being those with a long duration of action, which are as effective in a single dose within a few hours of delivery as are short-acting oestrogens given daily for 2 weeks. Quinestrol (Estrovis) is effective in a single dose of 4 mg and the effect is prolonged because the oestrogen is taken up by fat in the body and released over a prolonged period.

Androgens are effective a suppressing lactation but they occasionally give rise to a masculinising effect in the doses required. Mixtures of androgens and oestrogens have also been used but these appear to have no particular advantage.

The action of oestrogens in blocking puerperal lactation is peripheral and is not dependent on interference with prolactin secretion. In contrast, bromocriptine, a semi-synthetic ergot alkaloid, interferes with lactation by blocking prolactin secretion. Prolactin inhibitory factor is now thought to be dopamine. Bromocriptine stimulates dopamine receptors and thus inhibits the release of prolactin from the anterior pituitary gland. The treatment is strikingly effective in suppressing puerperal lactation, prolactin levels falling rapidly within a few hours (Varga et al 1972, Brun del Re et al 1973). Inhibition of lactation with bromocriptine has been evaluated in a large number of double blind trials and is superior to treatment with placebo, oestrogens and androgen/oestrogen preparations. It has the additional advantage over oestrogens that it does not alter blood clotting factors (Cooke et al 1972) and there have been no side effects reported with the small dose of bromocriptine which is effective. A typical course of treatment with bromocriptine is 2.5 mg on the first day followed by 2.5 mg twice daily for 2 weeks. Unlike oestrogen therapy, bromocriptine is effective even if the drug is administered after lactation is established (Brun del Re et al 1973).

Other drugs which have been used to suppress lactation include the antiserotonin agent metergoline (Delitala et al 1976) and pyridoxine (Carollo et al 1977); the anti-oestrogens clomiphene and tamoxifen (Masala et al 1978); and two other semisynthetic ergot derivatives, methysergide (Lancranjan et al 1979) and lisuride (De Cecco et al 1976). Most of these have been found to be less effective than bromocriptine, but lisuride may be a useful alternative.

**Summary**

No drug therapy can yet be recommended for women who appear to be lactating inadequately, though in some circumstances metoclopramide might be worth a trial. For the suppression of lactation, oestrogen therapy can now be regarded as superceded because of the increased risk of thrombo-embolism. The choice in lactation suppression is now between using no drug at all and using bromocriptine. Natural suppression without drug treatment may give rise to breast discomfort in some women and bromocriptine has been shown to abolish discomfort effectively. The use of bromocriptine is associated with two reservations. Most importantly, bromocriptine is a centrally acting dopaminergic drug interfering with the hypothalamic regulation of pituitary function. While this interference appears to be specific and reversible, the philosophy of using such a potent drug in a trivial self-limiting condition must be questioned. A second consideration is that the course of bromocriptine to suppress lactation is relatively expensive. Since bromocriptine is effective at suppressing breast discomfort at any time during the first week of lactation, it might be an effective plan to use it only for women with severe breast discomfort at the third or fourth day postpartum.

## DRUGS CONTAMINATING BREAST MILK

It is an obvious possibility that drugs given to a nursing woman may pass into her milk and adversely effect the suckling infant. Mothers are taking an increasing variety of drugs and, in particular, the immediate puerperium is a time of considerable drug use; analgesics, sedatives, antibiotics, anticoagulants and psychotropic drugs are frequently employed to cope with a variety of post-delivery problems.

Sixty-six per cent of drugs prescribed in an obstetric service were given to women in the immediate puerperium (Lewis et al 1980). Nursing mothers frequently ask their doctors if medicines they are taking can harm their infants. The clinician managing the patient obviously looks for precise information on a particular drug and is often irritated by his failure to find it in the literature.

In a recent World Health Organization bulletin (1979) it was reported that in the United States of America the Food and Drug Administration has recommended that drugs commonly used during labour or after delivery be labelled to provide information on any adverse effects on mother or child, the extent of drug excretion in human milk and effects on the breast fed infant. It is difficult to envisage this being implemented as there are few data on the extent to which drugs pass into human milk and little direct information can often be found about quite commonly used drugs in this respect. Although the literature on drugs in breast milk is quite extensive, much of it consists of case reports of isolated adverse events in breast feeding infants which might or might not have been due to the drugs their mothers were taking. Many pharmaceutical companies do not have information on the passage of drugs into breast milk and fall back on blanket statements such as 'The drug should only be used in nursing women if it is absolutely essential'. Paucity of data is not entirely due to lack of interest in the subject but more sinisterly to some idea that it is unethical in some way to investigate the passage of drugs into breast milk because it would involve experimentation on the neonate. It is fact perfectly possible to carry out transfer studies on drugs in lactating women who are not breast feeding their infants. Few such studies have been carried out.

## General principles

The risk to the breast fed infant of a particular drug being ingested by the mother is in many cases difficult to calculate. In the absence of precise information for any candidate drug the following following questions might be asked:

1. *Is the drug really needed by the mother?* This is probably the most crucial question that the clinician should ask himself. Obviously some treatments are essential. Many breast feeding women receive drugs by rote without any thought on the prescriber's part. For example, there is no justification for routinely treating women with sedatives in hospital, especially when they may cross into the breast milk and depress the infant.

2. *Would the drug do any harm if the infant did absorb it?* Unfortunately most drugs would be likely to have a harmful effect in

therapeutic doses. Anticoagulants and antimitotic drugs present an obvious hazard. Even such relatively innocuous substances as sedative, psychotropic drugs and anticonvulsants might sedate the infants sufficiently to interfere with efficient feeding. Sex hormones might upset the endocrine balance in the infant; neonatal hypothyroidism and cretinism can be produced by antithyroid drugs. Certain antibiotics are known to be toxic in the newborn. Sulphonamides can precipitate kernicterus even in mildly jaundiced infants, tetracycline can discolour the teeth and chloramphenicol, which is inadequately metabolised by neonates, accumulates and causes the so-called grey syndrome. Since neonates, particularly premature infants, have immature renal and hepatic function, their ability to eliminate drugs is limited. Thus the elimination half-time of most drugs is longer in neonates than in adults and this increases the potential toxicity as drug accumulation occurs.

3. *Would the drug be absorbed by the infant if it were present in the milk?* Unfortunately, any drugs sufficiently lipid soluble to enter the breast milk would probably be absorbed by the gastro-intestinal tract of the infant, so the answer to this question would be 'yes' for all the relevant drugs. In addition, the intestine of the newborn infant appears to permit absorption of undigested macromolecules (Walker and Hong 1973), so that the infant may become sensitised to trace amounts of drugs in milk.

4. *Does the drug get into the milk in significant quantities?* It is in this area that there are most difficulties, but the principles involved in the transfer of drugs into breast milk are now reasonably well established.

The dose that the infant receives depends on three factors: a] the plasma concentration of the drug in the mother; b] the extent of transfer of the drug from the mother's blood into the mother's milk; and c] the volume of milk that the infant consumes.

*The concentration of drug in the plasma* depends upon the pharmacokinetics of the drug in the mother. Most important is the volume of distribution of the drug. Fortunately, for most drugs the volume of distribution is high and hence the plasma concentration is relatively low.

*The extent of transfer of drug from mother's blood to milk* can be referred to as the milk to plasma ratio (M/P). Drugs absorbed by the mother reach mammary blood vessels via the general circulation and then have to traverse the mammary gland epithelium to reach the milk. Drugs may cross this barrier by two mechanisms: a] active transport b] passive diffusion.

Active transport differs from a passive process in that it exhibits selectivity, saturability and a requirement for energy. The transported substance is transferred against an electrochemical gradient; many organic acids and bases cross the renal tubule, choroid plexus and hepatic cells by this means. At present only thiouracil and iodine are thought to be secreted into breast milk by active transport. In the original study it was reported that the concentration of thiouracil in two samples of human milk was three times higher than that in whole blood taken at the same time (Williams et al 1944). Calculations based on a passive diffusion model, outlined below, predict milk concentrations less than half those in serum (Walker and Hong 1973). As most of the thiouracil in blood is present in the cells (Williams et al 1944) the 'milk to whole blood' ratio would be reduced still further, below 0.5. Hence, thiouracil is regarded as being actively transported into breast milk. In contrast, another antithyroid drug, propylthiouracil, has recently been shown to have maximum concentrations in milk only 10 per cent of the maximum serum level (Kampmann et al 1978, Low et al 1979), in full agreement with the calculations. Caution must continue concerning the use of thiouracil in breast feeding mothers, but not necessarily other antithyroid drugs, and doubt must remain about the thiouracil results in view of the small number of samples analysed.

The evidence for an active transport mechanisms for iodine is better documented. In 1952 it was shown that the concentration of radio-iodine in maternal milk, following an oral dose of 100 $\mu$Ci $^{131}$I, was sufficiently high to allow a sizeable uptake into the thyroid gland of the baby (Nurnberger and Lipscomb 1952). Other reports have shown that only free isotope is secreted into breast milk from in plasma at the same time (Miller and Weetch 1955, Weaver et al 1960). Most of the $^{131}$I is secreted in the first 24 hours and the percentage of the maternal dose received by the infant is roughly proportional to the amount of milk produced. In one case it was 23 per cent in 24 hours (Weaver et al 1960). More recently it has been shown that only free isotope is secreted into breast milk from $^{131}$I-labelled carriers such as albumin (Karjalainen et al 1971, Wyburn 1973). Under these circumstances the peak levels of $^{131}$I in milk are lower than if free isotope had been administered, and the peak levels are reached later, presumably because the carrier must first be degraded to release the iodine.

Most drugs appear to gain access to breast milk by passive diffusion. Non-electrolytes with a molecular weight under 200, such as ethanol, urea and antipyrine, enter milk by diffusion through the pores of the mammary gland epithelium. One of the criteria of passage by diffusion is that the concentrations of a drug at equilibrium are identical in the aqueous phases on either side of the membrane. In the case of ethanol, which is not bound to plasma protein, equal concentrations are produced in blood and milk (Kesäniemi 1974). It is interesting to note that although acetaldehyde is a non-electrolyte of lower molecular weight than ethanol, none could be detected

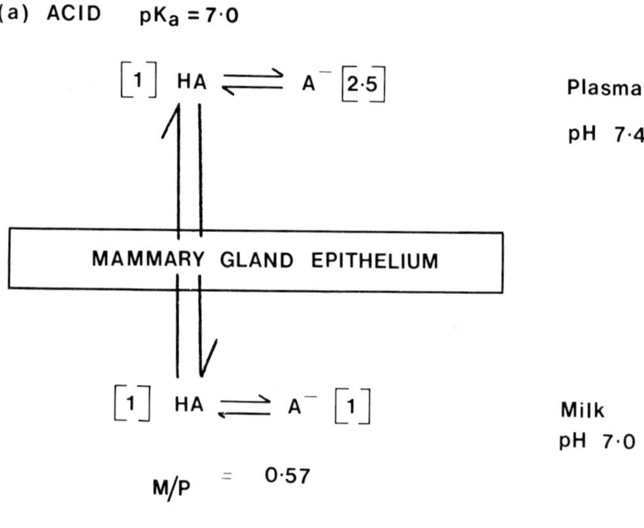


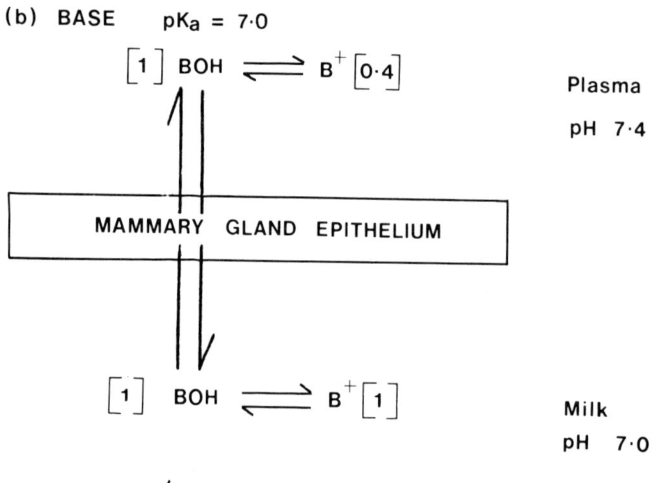


**Figure 14.1** Schematic representation of the distribution of a weak acid (a) and a weak base (b) across the mammary gland epithelium.

in milk, even though considerable amounts were measured in the blood (90 nmol/ml). This suggests that the mammary gland can exclude drugs just as it can concentrate them. The majority of drugs are weak acids or bases and exist in solution as a mixture of non-ionised and ionised species. Acidic drugs will dissociate into ions more in an alkaline medium than an acidic one, the reverse being the case for basic drugs. Non-ionised drugs cross the cellular barrier much better than ionised because the cell membrane possesses a highly polar phospholipid-protein structure. The non-ionised portion of a drug in blood diffuses passively into milk and at equilibrium the non-ionised concentrations are equal (Figure 14.1). As human milk usually has a more acidic pH than plasma Table 14.1 the dissociation of a drug differs in these two media and the total concentrations of drugs is unequal. As a general rule, weak acids achieve a lower concentration in milk than in plasma ($M/P \leqslant 1.0$) and weak bases achieve concentrations in milk which are similar to, or higher than, those in plasma ($M/P \geqslant 1.0$).

**Table 14.1** A comparison between the composition of human milk and plasma

| Constituent | Colostrum | Mature human milk | Plasma |
|---|---|---|---|
| pH | – | 6.7–7.4 | 7.4 |
| water (g/l) | 870 | 875 | 920 |
| carbohydrate (g/l) | 53 | 70 (lactose) | 0.8 (glucose) |
| fat (g/l) | 29 | 37 | 2 |
| protein (g/l) | | | |
| total | 58 | 12 | 70 |
| albumin | 12 | 3 | 45 |
| globulin | 11 | 2 | 25 |

This theoretical relationship can be expressed mathematically in the following derivation from the Henderson-Hasselbach equation:

$$\text{For acidic drugs: } \frac{C_m}{C_p} = \frac{1 + 10^{(pH_m - pK_a)}}{1 + 10^{(pH_p - pK_a)}} \cdot \frac{f_p}{f_m}$$

$$\text{For basic drugs: } \frac{C_m}{C_p} = \frac{1 + 10^{(pK_a - pH_m)}}{1 + 10^{(pK_a - pH_p)}} \cdot \frac{f_p}{f_m}$$

where $C_m$ = concentration of the drug in milk; $C_p$ = concentration of the drug in plasma = $pK_a$ = $pK_a$ of the drug; $pH_m$= milk pH; $pH_p$ = plasma pH; $f_m$ = fraction of drug unbound in milk; $f_p$ = fraction of drug unbound in plasma.

The $pK_a$ is a mathematical expression which corresponds to the pH at which the drug is 50 per cent dissociated, and is a constant for each particular drug. The two important variables are pH of milk ($pH_m$) and the protein binding of the drug ($f_m$ and $f_p$).

The normal pH of blood varies little and so can be regarded as constant at 7.4. In contrast, the pH of milk can vary significantly and could have an effect on the milk to plasma ratio. Many authors quote values of 6.8 and 7.0, but a more realistic value seems to be greater than 7.0. Pooled human breast milk gave a pH of 7.12 (Toh and Ho 1978) and pH measurements made on fresh milk from six women before and after feeds showed a slight rise in value from 7.27 to 7.38, with a range of values from 6.7 to 7.8 (Hall 1979). A more detailed study of milk pH is needed, particularly as values greater than 7.4 will reverse the milk to plasma ratios for acidic and basic drugs. The importance of this variation is highlighted by a comparison with saliva to plasma ratio. The same equations can be applied to this ratio as to milk, but saliva pH varies markedly according to its rate of production. Hence it is possible to predict plasma concentrations of drug by measurement in saliva when the drug is largely non-ionised at normal plasma pH (e.g. phenytoin and antipyrine); but this method is unreliable for ionised drugs (e.g. chlorpropramide and propranolol) because of the wide inter-individual variability of saliva pH (Mucklow et al 1978).

Many drugs are highly bound to plasma proteins and show a dynamic equilibrium between free and bound drug. The degree of protein binding is characteristic for any drug. For example, warfarin, the anticoagulant, is highly protein-bound in plasma (99 per cent), ampicillin is only weakly bound in plasma (20 per cent) and ethanol is not bound to protein at all. This is important because only the free (unbound) drug is available to diffuse into the milk. Thus protein binding reduces the amount of drug available for diffusion and affects the milk to plasma ratio. Once in the milk the drug may become bound to milk protein. Reference to Table 14.1 shows that the concentration of protein in mature milk is very much less than in plasma. Little is known about the drug-binding characteristics of milk proteins but drug-protein binding in milk is generally found to be much less than in plasma. Hence when the free concentrations of drug in milk and plasma are at equilibrium the total amount of drug in the plasma is greater because there is more drug attached to plasma protein than to milk protein. For a drug uniquely influenced by protein binding the ultrafiltrates of blood and milk would have the same drug concentration at equilibrium.

The protein content of milk remains fairly constant once mature milk is produced, but the fat content has been shown to vary significantly. The postpartum mammary secretion of colostrum (up to 1 week) is followed by a 2 to 3 week period of transitional milk secretion gradually leading to production of mature milk (Vorrherr 1974). Fat content increases in the transition from colostrum to mature milk (Table 14.1) and has been shown to increase markedly during the first 6 days postpartum, from 18 to 35 g/l (Lavric and Dolar 1976). Lipid content also exhibits a diurnal variation (Gunther and Starnier 1949) and increases within a feed (Hytten 1954). These variations will not alter the milk to plasma ratio directly as most drugs which can traverse the mammary gland epithelium must be lipid soluble and the drug dissolved in lipid is still un-ionised and therefore part of the equilibrium. It is important that the assay technique for the drug measures the lipid as well as the aqueous fraction, as the former can constitute a considerable, and variable, part of the total (Rasmussen 1966).

The process of diffusion, although passive, is usually rapid and for many drugs equilibrium between plasma and milk levels is achieved within minutes. Furthermore, diffusion is an equilibration process without any fixed direction and concentrations of drug in milk rise and fall, reflecting changes in plasma concentration. It might be thought that the amount of drug in milk would reflect the plasma concentration at the moment of production of the milk. In this way the milk already secreted into a cow's udder might form a reservoir with a fixed concentration of drug. This is not the case, for it has been shown experimentally that diffusion is a rapid enough process to allow equilibrium between blood and the secreted milk even when large quantities of milk are lying free in a reservoir (Rasmussen 1966). In the human breast, much less milk is produced between feeds so that there is not much reservoir milk in the ducts. Hence the concentrations of drug in milk ought to be related to the plasma concentration of the drug at the particular time that feeding takes place. Unfortunately this is not necessarily the case. Much of the work which developed these theoretical concepts was conducted on animals in which infusions maintained constant plasma concentrations of drug. Under clinical conditions plasma levels are not constant but are either rising or falling, depending on the route and interval of administration. The equilibrium between plasma and milk then seems to be delayed (Rasmussen 1966, Sisodia and Stowe 1964). During a period of falling plasma levels, the milk to plasma ratios were greater than the theoretical ratio, while during a period of rising plasma levels, the ratios were lower than the theoretical value. If the plasma levels rise or fall more rapidly than diffusion can take place then these results are expected, and milk can be

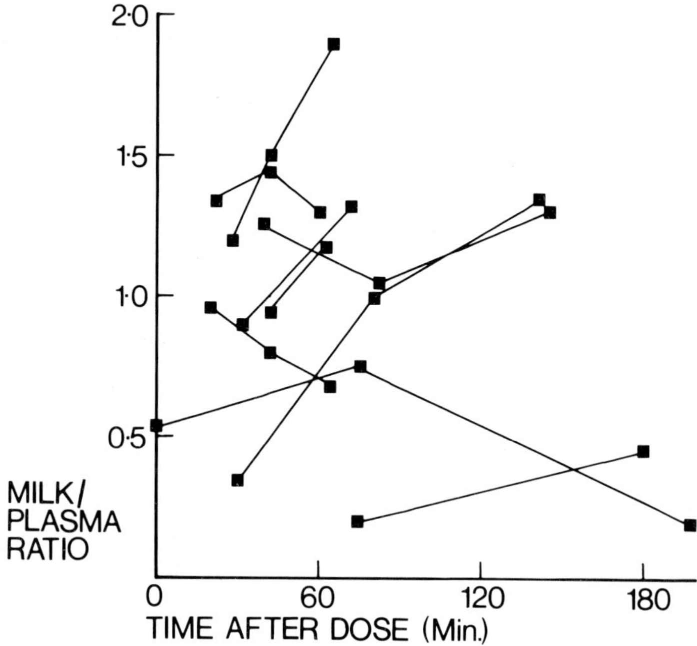


**Figure 14.2** Milk to plasma concentration ratios for paracetamol in 9 women following 1 g orally. Note the wide variation in the ratios and the lack of a consistent trend in ratios with time.

regarded as a pharmacokinetic 'deep compartment'. Intravenous injection of different sulphonamides showed differences in the rate of mammary excretion (Sisodia and Stowe 1964), and more recently theophylline (Yurchak and Jusko 1976), captopril (Devlin and Fleiss 1980) and salicylate (Berlin et al 1980) have also shown a delay between the attainment of peak plasma levels and peak milk levels. Work in this laboratory on paracetamol excretion in breast milk has shown that although the mean milk to plasma ratio obtained from 32 samples of milk was 1.0, which agrees with the theoretical value, the range was 0.2 to 1.9 and these ratios showed no consistent pattern in relation to rising or falling plasma levels (Figure 14.2). Other authors have noted variations in the milk to plasma ratio for a particular drug and so caution must be exercised when drawing conclusions about drug safety based on theoretical calculations calculations. Although much of the theory holds true for most drugs, we still do not entirely understand the effects of variations in, for example, milk pH, milk production rate and protein-binding.

*The volume of milk consumed by the infant* is important, as this, together with the concentration of the drug in milk, determines the quantity of drug consumed. There is an enormous individual variation, basically due to differences in mammary gland development (Hytten 1976), and it is difficult to assess the quantity accurately. At 1 week, the volume of milk at each feed was estimated at 20–45 ml, slowly increasing to 120–225 ml at 24 weeks (Holt 1972). The milk yield of 500 primiparae on the seventh day of lactation gave a mean of 400–500 ml (Hytten 1976), with a small percentage of the mothers producing as much as 1 litre per day. Any calculation of drug intake could thus be estimated by multiplying the mean milk concentration by 500–1000 ml. An important point is that colostrum, produced in the first few days post partum, is only secreted in amounts of 10–40 ml/day (Vorherr 1974). Although this represents a smaller intake, concentrations of drug in colostrum may be higher than predicted by calculation because of the difference in composition of colostrum compared to mature milk. This is an area worthy of particular study, as so many drugs are prescribed in the immediate puerperium.

## Specific drugs

The literature on adverse effects of drugs in breast milk is frequently incomplete, so that it is difficult to state with complete certainty that one particular drug is known to be free of hazard. Despite these reservations it would seem helpful to provide some tables on specific drugs. Table 14.2 lists drugs where some deleterious effect has been reported to arise in an infant whose mother was taking the drug. The drugs in Table 14.3 are those where too little information exists to say that the drug is completely without hazard. In Table 14.4 are listed drugs which seem to be without hazard for the breast feeding infant.

It may be helpful to discuss some classes of drugs in order to amplify these lists and in particular discuss those drugs often given to puerperal women. It is important to remember that the amounts of most drugs in breast milk are very small and undue alarm should

**Table 14.2** Drugs where deleterious effects have been reported —not safe for nursing mothers

| | |
|---|---|
| Amantadine | Lithium |
| Antineoplastic drugs | Phenindione |
| Chloramphenicol | Thiouracil |
| Ergot alkaloids | Any radiochemical |
| Iodine | |

**Table 14.3** Drugs where there is too little information to be categorical but some doubt remains as to their safety for use by nursing mothers.

| | |
|---|---|
| Anthraquinones | Nalidixic acid |
| Barbiturates (safe in low doses) | Oral contraceptives (safe in low doses) |
| Cimetidine | Phenylbutazone |
| Indomethacin | Reserpine |
| Isoniazid | Sulphonamides |
| Methydopa | Tetracycline |
| Metronidazole | Thiazide diuretics |

**Table 14.4** Drugs where no deleterious effect has been reported and which are probably safe for use by nursing mothers.

| | | |
|---|---|---|
| Alcohol | Erythromycin | Nitrofurantoin |
| Ampicillin | Folic acid | Paracetamol |
| Antihistamines | Frusemide | Penicillin |
| Caffeine | Gentamycin | Pentazocine |
| Carbamazepine | Guanethidine | Pethidine |
| Carbenicillin | Heparin | Phenothiazines |
| Cephaloridine | Heroin | Potassium iodide |
| Chloral | Imipramine | Propanthelene |
| Chlordiazepoxide | Iron | Quinine |
| Chloroquine | Kanamycin | Salicylates |
| Chlorpromazine | Lincomycin | Sodium fucidate |
| Codeine | Mefenamic acid | Streptomycin |
| Desipramine | Methylergometrine | Thyroxine |
| Dichloralphenazone | Morphine | Tolbutamide |
| Digoxin | Nitrazepam | Warfarin |

not be taken merely at the presence of a drug in milk. All other factors should be taken into consideration before discontinuing medication or breast feeding.

*Analgesics*

Although opiates can be detected in breast milk they are present in very small amounts and are thought to be unlikely to affect the infant (Anderson 1977, White 1977). It is of relevance to this that in the case of heroin addiction breast feeding alone is not considered sufficient to prevent withdrawal symptoms in the neonate, indicating that insufficient drug is transferred to have a pharmacological effect. Aspirin (Erickson and Oppenheim 1979) and paracetamol (Hurden, Harvey and Lewis, unpublished observations) may be used in the puerperium but indomethacin has been implicated in causing convulsions in a single case report (Eeg-Olofsson et al 1978), although no estimations of the drug were performed in either the mother or infant. Phenylbutazone is a potentially toxic substance which could not be detected in the milk of 20 women up to 3 hours after a 600 mg i.m. dose, but was found in low levels after a 750 mg i.m. dose (Knowles 1965). Caution is therefore advisable with this drug.

*Contraceptives*

The amount of progesterone or oestrogen transferred to milk is less than 1 per cent of the maternal dose, and low dose oral contraceptives are widely used in breast feeding women without any known toxicity. There are isolated case reports of two male infants developing gynaecomastia (Curtis 1964, Marriq and Oddo 1974) and several female infants were found to have proliferation of the vaginal epithelium (Lauritzen 1967), but the mothers were taking high dose oral contraceptive pills. The milk to plasma ratio for the depot contraceptive medroxyprogesterone was about 1.0, so that infants would again receive less than 1 per cent of the maternal dose (Saxena et al 1977, Koetsawang 1977).

*Anticoagulants*

There has been some controversy about anticoagulants and breast feeding. Heparin does not enter breast milk at all, as it is a high molecular weight mucopolysaccharide ionised at physiological pH. It is ineffective when administered orally. Warfarin does not seem to enter breast milk in sufficient amounts (Orme et al 1977), presumably because it is highly protein bound. Heparin and warfarin can safely be given to breast feeding women, warfarin being more convenient. Phenindione passes more readily into breast milk (Goguel 1970) and a breast fed infant whose mother was taking phenindione developed a severe haematoma after herniotomy at the age of 1 (Eckstein and Jack 1970). In view of the high incidence of hypersensitivity reactions to phenindione this drug should not be used in lactating women.

*Thyroid drugs*

As previously discussed, both thiouracil and iodine appear to be actively transported into milk (Williams et al 1944, Nurnberger and Lipscomb 1952, Miller and Weetch 1955, Weaver et al 1960), Karjalainen et al 1971, Wyburn 1973) and mothers requiring these drugs should not breast feed as their infants may develop hypothyroidism and goitre. If radioactive iodine is used, breast feeding should be stopped beforehand and up to 10 days afterwards (Karjalainen et al 1971, Wyburn 1973). More recently it has been demonstrated that less than 0.1 per cent of the maternal dose of propylchiouracil is found in breast milk (Kampmann et al 1978, Low et al 1979) and there were no changes in the thyroid parameters of a baby studied up to 5 months whose mother was receiving 200–300 mg of propylthiouracil daily. Thus antithyroid therapy should not be an absolute contraindication to breast feeding, providing the mother is on small doses of an antithyroid drug (propylthiouracil rather than carbimazole or methimazole) and the thyroid hormones of the baby are closely monitored.

There has been considerable discrepancy on the transfer of maternal thyroid hormones into milk. It now appears that human milk contains little or no $T_4$, whereas $T_3$ is detectable with a milk to plasma ratio of 0.1 (Varma et al 1978, Sato and Suzuki 1979). On the basis of these results human milk cannot be regarded as a useful source of thyroid hormones for the breast-fed baby, and the thyroid hormone content is not likely to mask hypothyroidism in the neonate.

*Antibiotics*

The penicillins and aminoglycoside antibiotics all pass into milk to a greater or lesser extent, but no adverse effects have been reported. In theory, it is possible for infants to become sensitised to the effect of penicillins and allergy might be produced. Again in theory, the aminoglycosides might cause ototoxicity in the infant, although this possibility is greatly reduced by their poor intestinal absorption. The level of metronidazole in milk is comparable to that in serum but the dose to the infant is quite low (Gray et al 1961). It is not known whether any adverse effect could be induced in babies.

All the sulphonamides are transferred to milk to a greater or lesser extent depending on their protein binding. These drugs may precipitate kernicterus in the jaundiced infant and one child with glucose-6-phosphate dehydrogenase deficiency developed haemolytic anaemia whilst the mother was taking sulphamethoxypyridazine (Hadley and Robin 1966).

Breast feeding is probably contraindicated during chloramphenicol treatment. Although the milk to plasma ratio is 0.5 and 50 per cent of the drug is present in milk as a metabolite that has no antibacterial activity (Havelka 1968), the drug may harm bone marrow and a number of adverse reactions in infants have been reported after feeding, including refusal of the breast and vomiting (Havelka and Fronkova 1972).

Tetracyclines theoretically cause mottling of the teeth if absorbed by the infant but are probably bound by the calcium in milk which will retard absorption (British Medical Journal 1969) and no adverse effects have been reported.

Nalidixic acid taken by the mother was suspected to be the cause of haemolytic anaemia in a suckling infant (Belton and Jones 1965) but the mother was uraemic and also taking amylobarbitone.

*Antihypertensive and thiazides*

Reserpine appears in breast milk but no adverse effects have been reported. Propranolol is also excreted but the amounts are unlikely to affect the infant (Bauer et al 1979). A report (Levitan and Marion 1973) stated that a maximal dose of 15 to 20 mg could be ingested by a nursing infant from a mother receiving a 40 mg oral dose of propranolol, but this was subsequently corrected to read 15–20 $\mu$g/24 h (Anderson and Salter 1976). Thiazide diuretics appear in breast milk but levels are probably insignificant (Werthmann and Kress 1972).

*Anticonvulsants and sedative-hypnotics*

Nursing mothers can generally take anticonvulsant doses of barbituates without affecting the infant. Caution should be exercised when the mother is taking barbiturates over a long period or in excessive amounts. Usually single high doses of barbiturates have more potential for causing infant drowsiness than multiple small doses (Anderson 1977). One child developed methaemoglobinaemia while his mother was taking large doses of phenobarbitone and phenytoin (Finch et al 1954).

Pharmacologically insignificant amounts of carbamazepine have been detected in breast milk (Pynnönen et al 1977, Niebyl et al 1979). Diazepam should be avoided as in one report an infant became lethargic and lost weight until breast feeding stopped (Patrick et al 1972) and other authors have highlighted the risk of drug accumulation and the production of neonatal jaundice (Erkkola and Kanto 1972). Nitrazepam appears in breast milk at concentrations of 50 to 100 ng/ml after daily doses of 5–10 mg and is unlikely to produce any toxic effects in the child (Rieder and Wendt 1973).

Advice on chlorpromazine is conflicting, the levels in milk being variously estimated as negligible (Blacker et al 1962) or significant (Citterio 1964). More recently Wiles et al (1978) reported no clear or consistent relationship between plasma and milk levels. Apart from one infant appearing drowsy and lethargic (Wiles et al 1978) no other adverse effects have been reported.

Lithium enters breast milk with a milk to plasma ratio between

0.3 and 0.5 (Schou and Amdisen 1973). As the drug is completely absorbed from the gastrointestinal tract and toxic effects are likely, breast feeding is contraindicated (Schou and Amdisen 1973, Tunnessen and Hertz 1972, Ananth 1978).

The tricyclic antidepressants imipramine, desipramine and amitriptyline are all transferred to milk in insignificant amounts.

*Miscellaneous drugs*

The milk to plasma ratio for digoxin is about 0.9 (Loughnan 1978, Finley et al 1979) but infant exposure is low and breast feeding may safely be permitted.

The data on antineoplastic drugs is scarce. Cyclophosphamide has been detected in milk, but not quantitated (Wiernick and Duncan 1971) and methotrexate has a milk to plasma ratio of less than 0.1 (Johns et al 1972). Although some authors consider it safe to breast feed, the possible long term effects of these compounds would suggest otherwise.

Ergot alkaloids enter breast milk, produce symptoms in suckling infants (Illingworth 1953) and should be avoided. Indeed many ergot derivatives, such as bromocriptine, can suppress lactation. Ergometrine is used as an oxytocic after delivery but has not been measured in breast milk. In contrast, methylergometrine, a semisynthetic ergot alkaloid used in the same way, has been shown to have a milk to plasma ratio of about 0.3 and the levels were not considered harmful to the infant (Erkkola et al 1978), particularly in short-term use.

With the possible exception of anthraquinone derivatives, laxatives do not cause purgation in the breast fed infant. Even anthraquinones have not been clearly shown to have an effect on the infant's bowel motility (Vorrherr 1974).

Cimetidine gave highly variable milk to plasma ratios in one patient after chronic doses (Somogyi and Gugler 1979), values being several times higher than that predicted by calculation. These results may have been due to a 'lag' in attaining equilibrium between milk and plasma, rather than an active secretory process, but the drug should be used with caution until further studies have been completed.

The methylxanthines, theophylline (Yurchak and Jusko 1976), theobromine (Resman et al 1977) and caffeine (Tyrala and Dodson 1979), are all excreted in low amounts in milk and no adverse effects have been shown.

A moderate amount of alcohol ingestion by the nursing mother does not affect the child. Common sense should dictate that excessive drinking is to be avoided (Binkiewitz et al 1978) and in any event high levels of alcohol inhibit the milk ejection reflex (Cobo 1973).

Similarly, moderate smoking is permissible. The infant is probably in more danger from inhaled cigarette smoke than from consuming milk containing small quantities of nicotine, a compound which is not readily absorbed from the gastrointestinal tract. Heavy smoking has also been suggested to interfere with milk supply.

### *Environmental agents*

Although such compounds as insecticides do not come strictly under the heading of drugs, nevertheless, they can lead to toxic effects in breast fed infants. The level of such agents consumed by mothers is, of course, beyond their control and also subject to wide geographical variation. A few examples will illustrate the problems which can and do arise, albeit rarely. In Turkey, breast fed infants were poisoned and died after the mother had consumed wheat treated with the fungicidal agent hexachlorobenzene (Knowles 1974). In Iraq infants were found to be ingesting mercury from the mother's milk, following the consumption of wheat treated with a methyl mercury fungicide (Clarkson et al 1974, Amin-Zaki et al 1974) and mercury contaminated fish gave rise to toxic effects in Japan (Knowles 1974). It is not known what effect the extremely high levels of DDT found in breast milk will have on the infants concerned in central and southern America (Olzynska-Marays 1978).

## CONCLUSION

Not unreasonably, pharmaceutical companies complain that the merest hint of an adverse effect on a child from a drug present in breast milk is quickly accepted as an irrefutable fact, whilst claims that the same drug produces a miracle cure are treated with scepticism. We should remind ourselves that the number of reports which clearly implicate a drug present in breast milk as causing toxicity in an infant is very small. Although many drugs are present in milk in concentrations similar to, or greater than, the concentrations in maternal plasma, the quantity of drug ingested by the child is small and generally insignificant. With the exception of those drugs listed in Table 14.2 there is far less cause for concern than some previous reviewers of the subject would have us believe.

## REFERENCES

Amin-Zaki L, Elhassani S, Majeed M A, Carkson T W, Doherty R A, Greenwood M R 1974 Studies of infants postnatally exposed to methylmercury. Journal of Pediatrics 85: 81–84

Ananth J 1978 Side effects in the neonate from psychotropic agents excreted through breast-feeding. American Journal of Psychiatry 135: 801–805

Anderson P O 1977 Drugs and breast feeding – a review. Drug Intelligence and Clinical Pharmacy 11: 208–223

Anderson P O, Salter F J 1976 Propranolol therapy during pregnancy and lactation. American Journal of Cardiology 37: 325

Bauer J H, Page B, Zajicek J, Groshing T 1979 Propranolol in human plasma and breast milk. American Journal of Cardiology 43: 860–862

Belton E M, Jones R V 1965 Haemolytic anaemia due to nalidixic acid. Lancet ii: 691

Berlin C M, Pascuzzi M J, Jaffe S J, 1980 Excretion of salicylate in human milk. Journal of Clinical Pharmacology and Therapeutics 27: 245–246

Binkiewicz H, Robinson M J, Senior B 1978 Pseudo-Cushing syndrome caused by alcohol in breast milk. Journal of Pediatrics 93: 965–967

Blacker K H, Weinstein B J, Ellman G G 1962 Mother's milk and chlorpromazine. American Journal of Psychiatry 119: 178–179

British Medical Journal 1969 Tetracycline in breast milk. British Medical Journal iv: 791

Brun del Re R, del Pozo E, de Grandi P, Friesen H, Hinselmann M, Wyss H 1973 Prolactin inhibition and suppression of puerperal lactation by a Bromocryptine (CB 154) A comparison with oestrogen. Obstetrics and Gynecology 41: 884–890

Canales E S, Lasso P, Murrieta S, Fonseca E, Soria J, Zarate, A 1977 Feasibility of suppressing and reinitiating lactation in women with premature infants. American Journal of Obstetrics and Gynecology 128: 695–697

Carollo F, Barreca P, Palisi F 1977 Inhibition of lactation and lowering of plasma prolactin by administration of pyridoxine. Clinical Teratology 81: 213–219

Citterio C 1964 Identification and determination of phenothiazine derivatives in milk. Neuropsychiatry 20: 141–143

Clarkson T W, Doherty R A, Greenwood M 1974 Intrauterine methylmercury poisoning in Iraq. Pediatrics 54: 587–595

Cobo E 1973 Effect of different doses of ethanol on the milk-ejecting reflex in lactating women. American Journal of Obstetrics and Gynecology 115: 817–821

Cooke I, Foley M, Lenton E et al 1972 The treatment of puerperal lactation with bromocriptine. Postgraduate Medical Journal 52 (supplement 1): 75–80

Curtis E M 1964 Oral contraceptive feminization of a normal male infant. Obstetrics and Gynecology 23: 295–296

Daniel D G, Campbell H, Turnbull, A C 1967 Puerperal thrombo-embolism and suppression of lactation. Lancet ii: 287–289

De Cecco L, Venturini P L, Ragni N, Rossato P, Maganza C, Gaggero G 1976 Effect of lisuride on inhibition of lactation and serum prolactin. British Journal of Obstetrics and Gynaecology 86: 905–908

Delitala G, Masala A, Lodico G, Milia S 1976 Inhibition of puerperal lactation; comparison of metergoline, an antiserotonin agent, with bromocriptine, a dopamine agonist. Studi Sassaresi 54: 3

Devlin R G, Fleiss P M 1980 Selective resistance to the passage of captopril into human milk. Journal of Clinical Pharmacology and Therapeutics 27: 250

Eckstein H B, Jack B 1970 Breast feeding and anticoagulant therapy. Lancet i: 672–673

Eeg-Olofsson O, Malmros I, Elwin C E, Steen B 1978 Convulsions in a breast-fed infant after maternal indomethacin. Lancet ii: 215

Erickson S H, Oppenheim G L 1979 Aspirin in breast milk. Journal of Family Practice 8: 189–190

Erkkola R, Kanto J 1972 Diazepam and breast-feeding. Lancet i: 1235–1236

Erkkola R, Kanto J, Allonen H, Kelimola T, Mäntylä R 1978 Excretion of methylergometrine (methylergonovine) into the human breast milk. International Journal of Clinical Pharmacology, Therapy and Toxicology 16: 579–580

Finch E, Lorber J 1954 Methaemoglobinaemia in the newborn probably due to phenytoin excreted in human milk. Journal of Obstetrics and Gynaecology of the British Empire 61: 833–834

Finley J P, Waxman M B, Wong P Y, Lickrish G M 1979 Digoxin excretion in human milk (letter). Journal of Pediatrics 94: 339–340

Foss G L, Phillips P 1938 The suppression of lactation by oral oestrogen therapy. British Medical Journal ii: 887–890

Goguel M 1970 Therapeutique anticoagulante et allaitement: Etude du passage de la phenyl-2-dioxo-1, 3-indane dans le lait maternel. Revue Française de Gynécologie et d'Obstétrique 65: 409–412

Gray M S, Kane P O, Squires S 1961 Further observations on metronidazole (Flagyl). British Journal of Venereal Diseases 37: 278–279

Gunther M, Starnier J E 1949 Diurnal variation in the fat content of breast milk. Lancet ii: 235–237

Guzman V, Toscano G, Canales E S, Zarate A 1979 Improvement of defective lactation by using oral metoclopramide. Acta obstetricia et gynecologica Scandinavica 58: 53–55

Hadley J D, Robin H 1966 'Late' neonatal jaundice following maternal treatment with sulphamethoxypyridazine. Pediatrics 37: 855–856

Hall B 1979 Uniformity of human milk. American Journal of Clinical Nutrition 32: 304–312

Hall D M, Kay G 1977 Effect of thyrotophin-releasing factor on lactation. British Medical Journal i: 777

Havelka J 1968 Excretion of chloramphenicol in human milk. Chemotherapy 13: 204–211

Havelka J, Frankova A 1972 Study of side effects of maternal chloramphenicol therapy in newborns. Československá Pediatrie 21: 31–33

Holt L E 1972 Feeding techniques and diets. In: Barnett H L (editor) Pediatrics, 5th edition. Meredith, New York

Hytten F E 1954 Clinical and chemical studies in human lactation. British Medical Journal i: 175–182

Hytten F E 1976 The physiology of lactation. Journal of Human Nutrition 30: 225–232

Illingworth R S 1953 Abnormal substances excreted in human milk. Practitioner 171: 533–538

Johns D G, Rutherford L D, Leighton P C, Vogel C L 1972 Secretion of methotrexate into human milk. American Journal of Obstetrics and Gynecology 112: 978–980.

Kampmann J P, Johansen K, Hansen J M, Helweg J 1978 Propylthiouracil in human milk. Lancet i: 736–738

Karajalainen P, Penttila M, Pystynen P 1971 The amount and form of radioactivity in human milk after lung scanning, renography and placental localization by $I^{131}$ labelled tracers. Acta obstetricia et gynecologica Scandinavica 50: 357–361

Kesäniemi Y A 1974 Ethanol and acetaldehyde in the milk and peripheral blood of lactating women after ethanol administration. Journal of Obstetrics and Gynaecology of the British Commonwealth. 81: 84–86

Knowles J A 1965 Excretion of drugs in milk — a review. Journal of Pediatrics 65: 1068–1082

Knowles J A 1974 Breast milk: a source of more than nutrition for the neonate. Clinical Toxicology 7: 69–82

Koetsawang S 1977 Injected long-acting medroxyprogesterone acetate effect on human lactation and concentrations in milk. Journal of the Medical Association of Thailand. 60: 57–80

Lancranjan I, Del Pozo E, Picciolini E, D'Antona N, Genazzani A R 1979 Effect of two serotonin antagonists on prolactin release induced by breast stimulation in postpartum women. Hormone Research 10: 14–19

Lauritzen C 1967 On endocrine effects of oral contraceptives. Acta endocrinologica 124 (supplement): 87–100

Lavric M, Dolar J 1976 Human milk—variations in lactose, potassium, sodium and total lipid concentrations and in fatty acids composition of lactating women in early puerperium. Jugoslavenska Ginekologija i Opstetricija 16: 203–207.

Levitan A A, Manion J C 1973 Propranolol therapy during pregnancy and lactation. American Journal of Cardiology 32: 247

Lewis P J, Boylan P, Bulpitt C J 1980 An audit of prescribing in an obstetric service. British Journal of Obstetrics and Gynaecology 87: 1043–1045

Lewis P J, Devenish C, Khan C 1980 Controlled trial of metoclopramide in the initiation of breast feeding. British Journal of Clinical Pharmacology 9: 217–219

Loughnan P M 1978 Digoxin excretion in human breast milk. Journal of Pediatrics 92: 1019–1020

Low L C, Lang J, Alexander W D 1979 Excretion of carbimazole and propylthiouracil in breast milk. Lancet ii: 1011

McNeilly A S, Thorner M O, Volans G, Besser, G M 1974 Metoclopramide and prolactin. British Medical Journal ii: 729

Marriq P, Oddo G 1974 La gynecomastie induite chez le nouveau-né par le lait maternel? Nouveau Presse Médicale 3: 2579

Masala A, Delitala G, Lodico G, Stoppelli I, Alagna A, Devilla L 1978 Inhibition of lactation and inhibition of prolactin release after mechanical breast stimulation in puerperal women given tamoxifen or placebo. British Journal of Obstetrics and Gynaecology 85: 134–137

Miller H, Weetch R S 1955 The excretion of radioactive iodine in human milk. Lancet ii: 1013

Mucklow J C, Bending M R, Kahn G C, Dollery C T 1978 Drug concentration in saliva. Clinical Pharmacology and Therapeutics 24: 563–570

Niebyl J R, Blake D A, Freeman J M, Luff R D 1979 Carbamazepine levels in pregnancy and lactation. Obstetrics and Gynecology 53: 139–140

Nurnberger C E, Lipscomb A 1952 Transmission of radioiodine ($I^{131}$) to infants through human maternal milk. Journal of the American Medical Association 150: 1398–1400

Olszyna-Marzys A D 1978 Contaminants in human milk. Acta paediatrica Scandinavica 67: 571–576

Orme M L, Lewis P J, Serlin M J, Sibeon R, Baty J D, Breckenridge A M 1977 Can mothers given warfarin breast-feed their infants? British Medical Journal i: 1564–1565

Patrick M J, Tilstone W J, Reavey P 1972 Diazepam and breast feeding. Lancet i: 542–543

Pynnönen S, Kanto J, Sillanpäa M, Erkkola R 1977 Carbamazepine placental transport, tissue concentration in foetus and newborn, level in milk. Acta pharmacologica et toxicologica 41: 244–253

Rasmussen F 1966 Studies on the mammary excretion and absorption of drugs. Mortensen, Copenhagen

Resman B H, Blumenthal H P, Jusko W J 1977 Breast milk distribution of theobromine from chocolate. Journal of Pediatrics 91: 477–480

Rieder J, Wendt G 1973 Pharmacokinetics and metabolism of the hypnotic nitrazepam. In: Garattini S (editor) The benzodiazepines. Raven Press, New York, pp 99–127

Rigg L A, Lein A, Yen S S C 1977 Pattern of increase in circulating prolactin levels during human gestation. American Journal of Obstetrics and Gynecology 129: 453–456

Sato T, Suzuki Y 1979 Presence of triiodothyronine, no detectable thyroxine and reverse triiodothyronine in human milk. Endocrinologia Japonica 26: 507–513

Saxena B N, Shrimanker K, Grudzinskas J D 1977 Levels of contraceptive steroids in breast milk and plasma of lactating women. Contraception 16: 605–613

Schou M, Amdisen A 1973 Lithium and pregnancy. III Lithium ingestion by children breast-fed by women on lithium treatment. British Medical Journal ii: 138

Sisodia C S, Stowe C W 1964 The mechanism of drug secretion in bovine milk. Annals of the New York Academy of Sciences 111: 650–661

Somogyi A, Gugler R 1979 Cimetidine excretion into breast milk. British Journal of Clinical Pharmacology 7: 627–629

Sonson P L R 1975 Metoclopramide and breast feeding. British Medical Journal i: 512

Toh C C, Ho N K 1978 pH, titratable acidity and osmolality of human breast milk and some infant milk formulae. Journal of the Singapore Paediatric Society 20: 88–92

Tunnessen W W, Hertz C G 1972 Toxic effects of lithium in newborn infants: A commentary. Journal of Pediatrics 81: 804–807

Tyrala E E, Dodson W E 1979 Caffeine secretion into breast milk. Archives of Diseases in Childhood 54: 787–789

Tyson J E, Ewang P, Guyda H, Reieson H G 1972 Studies of prolactin secretion in human pregnancy. American Journal of Obstetrics and Gynecology 113: 14–20

Tyson J E, Khojandi M, Huth J, Andreassen B 1975 The influence of prolactin secretion on human lactation. Journal of Clinical Endocrinology and Metabolism 40: 764–773

Tyson J F, Perez A, Zanartu J 1976 Human lactational response to oral thyrotropin-releasing hormone. Journal of Clinical Endocrinology and Metabolism 43: 760768

Varga L, Lutterbeck P M, Pryor J S, Wenner R, Erb H 1972 Suppression of puerperal lactation with an ergot alkaloid; a double blind study. British Medical Journal ii: 743–744

Varma S K, Collins M, Row A, Haller W S, Varma K 1978 Thyroxine, tri-iodothyronine and reverse tri-iodothyronine concentrations in human milk. Journal of Pediatrics 93: 803–806

Vorrherr H 1974 The breast: Morphology, physiology and lactation. Academic Press, New York

Walker W A, Hong R 1973 Immunology of the gastrointestinal tract: Part I. Journal of Pediatrics 83: 517–530

Weaver J C, Kamm M L, Dobson R L 1960 Excretion of radioiodine in human milk. Journal of the American Medical Association 173: 872–875

Werthmann M W, Krees S V 1972 Excretion of chlorothiazide in human breast milk. Journal of Pediatrics 81: 781–783

Whichlow M J 1979 Breast feeding in Cambridge, England: factors affecting the mother's milk supply. Journal of Advanced Nursing 4: 253–261

White M 1977 Breastfeeding and drugs in human milk. La Leche League International, Illinois

Wiernick P H, Duncan J H 1971 Cyclophosphamide in human milk. Lancet i: 912

Wiles D H, Orr M W, Kolakowska T 1978 Chlorpromazine levels in plasma and milk of nursing mothers. British Journal of Clinical Pharmacology 5: 272–273

Williams R H, Kay G A, Jandorf B J 1944 Thiouracil. Its absorption, distribution and excretion. Journal of Clinical Investigation 23: 613–627

World Health Organization 1979 Drug information bulletin. Geneva, July–September

Wyburn J R 1973 Human breast milk excretion of radionuclides following adminstration of radiopharmaceuticals. Journal of Nuclear Medicine 14: 115–117

Yurchak A M, Jusko W J 1976 Theophylline scretion into breast milk. Pediatrics 57: 518–520

Zanartu J, Aguilera E, Jimerez J 1975 Role of synthetic hypothalamic prolactin releasing hormone and of some progestogens in stimulating and maintainging post-partum lactation. Revista médica de Chile 103: 699–706

Zarate A, Villabos E, Canales E S, Soria J, Arcovedo F, MacGregor C 1976 The effect of oral administration of thyrotropin releasing hormone on lactation. Journal of Clinical Endocrinology and Metabolism 43: 301–305

# Index